DIABETIC COOKING

FOR BEGINNERS!

Easy and tasty meals
appropriate for a diabetes diet

pi

Publications International, Ltd.

All recipes and recipe photographs copyright © Publications International, Ltd.

Pictured on the front cover: Farro, Chickpea & Spinach Salad (*page 78*).

Pictured on the back cover (*clockwise from top left*): Ham and Vegetable Omelet (*page 34*), Southwestern Tuna Salad (*page 60*), Orange Chicken (*page 122*), Yogurt "Custard" with Blueberries (*page 180*), and Peppy Snack Mix (*page 150*).

ISBN: 978-1-64030-727-8

Manufactured in China.

8 7 6 5 4 3 2 1

Note: This publication is only intended to provide general information. The information is specifically not intended to be a substitute for medical diagnosis or treatment by your physician or other health care professional. You should always consult your own physician or other health care professionals about any medical questions, diagnosis, or treatment. (Products vary among manufacturers. Please check labels carefully to confirm nutritional values.)

The information obtained by you from this book should not be relied upon for any personal, nutritional, or medical decision. You should consult an appropriate professional for specific advice tailored to your specific situation. PIL makes no representations or warranties, express or implied, with respect to your use of this information.

In no event shall PIL, its affiliates or advertisers be liable for any direct, indirect, punitive, incidental, special, or consequential damages, or any damages whatsoever including, without limitation, damages for personal injury, death, damage to property, or loss of profits, arising out of or in any way connected with the use of any of the above-referenced information or otherwise arising out of the use of this book.

WARNING: Food preparation, baking and cooking involve inherent dangers: misuse of electric products, sharp electric tools, boiling water, hot stoves, allergic reactions, foodborne illnesses and the like, pose numerous potential risks. Publications International, Ltd. (PIL) assumes no responsibility or liability for any damages you may experience as a result of following recipes, instructions, tips or advice in this publication.

While we hope this publication helps you find new ways to eat delicious foods, you may not always achieve the results desired due to variations in ingredients, cooking temperatures, typos, errors, omissions, or individual cooking abilities.

Let's get social!

 @Publications_International

 @PublicationsInternational

www.pilcookbooks.com

CONTENTS

KEY WORDS

GLUCOSE

Most of the sugar in your bloodstream is the kind called glucose. Glucose's main job is to supply the body's cells with energy. It's a quickly available fuel used by nearly all tissues in the body, and it's the only fuel your brain and nerves can use.

INSULIN

Insulin plays a major role in allowing the body's cells to take in proteins, fatty acids, and glucose. Insulin is like a key that opens a door to the body's cells, so the nutrients needed by the cells can get inside.

WHAT IS DIABETES?

Millions of people today either may have diabetes or are at risk for getting diabetes. Although there is currently no cure for the disease, it is very treatable. You can easily live a long and healthy life by understanding diabetes and taking care of yourself.

To get the most from the latest advances in diabetes care, you need to understand just what it means to have diabetes. A good place to start is learning how the body uses fuel and how that process goes awry in diabetes.

EDUCATING YOURSELF

Even if you've only recently been diagnosed with diabetes, you've probably already heard the word glucose. It's an important player in the body and in diabetes. In your bloodstream, circulating to all your body parts, is sugar. Most of the sugar in your bloodstream is the kind called glucose. Glucose's main job is to supply the body's cells with energy. Glucose is a quickly available fuel used by nearly all tissues in the body, and it's the only fuel your brain and nerves can use. The brain can survive without glucose for only a short time. Therefore, your brain directs your body to protect your glucose level, making sure it doesn't fall too low. It does this by increasing the production of certain hormones. These hormones cause the liver to release its stored-up sugar into the bloodstream. So, when people talk about blood sugar, they are really talking about glucose.

The glucose in your body comes from three major nutrients: fat, protein, and carbohydrate. About 10 percent of the fat and 50 percent of the protein you eat is eventually converted into glucose (the rest is used for other purposes or stored in the body's fat cells), but nearly 100 percent of the carbohydrate you eat is broken down into glucose. Chewing and swallowing begin the digestive process of breaking down starches and larger sugar molecules into glucose. The enzymes in your mouth and your intestines complete the breakdown. The glucose is then absorbed into the bloodstream and travels throughout the body. That's when the pancreas plays a vital role.

The pancreas is a fist-size organ just behind your stomach. One of its jobs is to make enzymes for food digestion. But, the pancreas also plays another important role. It contains small groups of cells, the islets of Langerhans, that make hormones, which are released into your bloodstream. Some 80 percent of these islet cells are called "beta" cells that make two hormones: amylin and insulin. Amylin plays a secondary role in regulating appetite and the rate of digestion. Insulin plays a major role in allowing the body's cells to take in proteins, fatty acids, and glucose. Insulin is like a key that opens a door to the body's cells, so the nutrients needed by the cells can get inside. When a person who does not have diabetes eats any food, their blood glucose level rises. The beta cells detect this rise and release more insulin. The insulin goes to the liver, telling the liver to make less glucose. It also helps the liver, muscle, and fat cells to take up more glucose. This allows nutrients from the recently eaten food to enter and "feed" the body's cells, it keeps blood glucose from rising too high even after eating, and it allows the glucose level to return to a normal, healthy range quickly. When we go many hours without eating, such as between meals or during sleep, the insulin levels fall, causing the liver to make more glucose to provide energy for the brain, heart, lungs, etc, until the next meal.

In a person with diabetes, this process doesn't work properly. Either the beta cells have lost the ability to produce insulin or the insulin does not do its job as well as it should. As a result, the amount of glucose in the blood rises and the body's cells become deprived of the fuel they need.

TYPES

T-1 DIABETES
Affects about 5 percent of all people with diabetes. May also be called insulin-dependent diabetes, due to insulin (via injections or an insulin pump) being required to not only control blood glucose, but to stay alive.

T-2 DIABETES
Most common form of diabetes. The cause appears to be resistance to insulin's action compounded by a deficiency of insulin secretion.

GESTATIONAL
Diagnosed for the first time during pregnancy. It occurs in about 3 percent of all pregnancies. Women who have had gestational diabetes have a significantly greater chance of developing diabetes later in life.

DIFFERENT TYPES OF DIABETES

There are three major types of diabetes: type 1 diabetes, type 2 diabetes, and gestational diabetes. Each type requires a different type of treatment.

TYPE 1 DIABETES

This type affects about 5 percent of all people with diabetes. It is sometimes referred to as juvenile diabetes, because there is a higher rate of diagnosis in children, but people of any age can develop type 1 diabetes. It may also be called insulin-dependent diabetes, because those with type 1 diabetes require insulin (via injections or an insulin pump) to not only control their blood glucose, but to stay alive.

TYPE 2 DIABETES

Type 2 diabetes is the most common form of diabetes. It is estimated that up to 90 percent of the people who have diabetes have type 2. The cause appears to be resistance to insulin's action compounded by a deficiency of insulin secretion.

People with type 2 diabetes are usually over age 35, are overweight, and have a family history of type 2 diabetes. Type 2 diabetes actually begins years before diagnosis, as an increasing resistance to insulin. This increasing resistance is the result of genetics, weight gain (especially abdominal fat), decreased activity, and aging. The major site of insulin resistance is the muscle tissue, which normally burns up the majority of the glucose in the bloodstream. When insulin has a difficult time "opening doors" on the body's cells, the pancreas tries to compensate by making more and more insulin. For some people, the pancreas is eventually unable to keep up with the increased workload. Blood glucose levels rise above normal after meals, and fasting glucose levels begin to remain above normal, too. Ironically, very high glucose levels can damage the beta cells, a condition called glucose toxicity. This further accelerates the breakdown of the pancreas' ability to control blood sugar levels. When glucose rises high enough to produce symptoms (excessive thirst, frequent urination, wounds that don't heal, for example), or when a complication such as a heart attack, stroke, visual disturbance, infection, numbness, or serious gum disease is treated, the diagnosis of type 2 diabetes is often made.

GESTATIONAL DIABETES

Gestational diabetes is diagnosed for the first time during pregnancy. It occurs in about 3 percent of all pregnancies. Gestational diabetes is diagnosed using a 3-hour glucose tolerance test. If any two of the glucose readings during the test exceed the upper limits of normal, the diagnosis is made. Rarely are the glucose levels high enough to harm the mother. The problem is the mother's blood. Extra glucose flows to the developing baby, which then produces extra insulin. This, in turn, causes the baby to grow too quickly, resulting in a difficult labor and delivery.

Throughout the pregnancy, the mother's insulin resistance and glucose levels increase, right up to delivery. In 97 percent of cases, the mother's glucose levels promptly return to normal after delivery. Many women with gestational diabetes can control their glucose levels during pregnancy through diet and exercise. Some, however, require insulin to keep glucose levels within a healthy range for the fetus.

Women who have had gestational diabetes have a significantly greater chance of developing diabetes later in life. Studies have shown that weight control and increased physical activity reduce the risk of future diabetes by as much as 50 percent.

YOUR DIABETES TOOL KIT

A diagnosis of diabetes can be disheartening, but there is plenty of good news. These days, you have many diabetes tools to help you keep your blood sugar under tight control and ward off the frightening complications. You simply need to understand how to apply them to your best advantage and to commit yourself to using them faithfully.

MONITORING YOUR GLUCOSE

Blood glucose monitoring is a vital part of the diabetes management process, and frequent self-monitoring is a key to successful care. By checking your glucose, you get a precise measurement of what your blood glucose level is so you can adjust your food, medication, or activity level accordingly. Knowing your glucose level also lets you see if your previous food, medication, or activity level brought your glucose to a desired range. It means for greater freedom to participate in any activities you choose and, therefore, far greater control over your life. The blood glucose values are like clues in a mystery novel. The more clues you have, the greater your ability to solve the mystery. Of course, the opposite can be true as well. The less you check, the fewer clues you have and the more your diabetes remains a mystery to both you and your diabetes care team.

Checking your blood glucose on a regular basis allows you to know the ongoing status of your diabetes and will help you learn more about it and your body. Checking multiple times each day will give you even more information, helping you understand blood glucose patterns that occur when you eat certain foods and take specific medication doses, as well as how these are connected to your level of activity and stressors at home or work. Frequent checking also ensures that you can catch high or low levels quickly and respond to them with appropriate adjustments.

IMPORTANT

GLUCOSE MONITORING IS A MUST

It gives a precise measurement of what your blood glucose level is so you can adjust your food, medication, or activity level accordingly.

Checking your levels multiple times each day will give you even more information, helping you understand blood glucose patterns that occur when you eat certain foods and take specific medication doses, as well as how these are connected to your level of activity and stressors at home or work.

EATING FOR BETTER CONTROL

When you learned you had diabetes, you may have assumed you'd have to go on a special, restrictive diet. Perhaps you'd heard of people with diabetes who had to give up every food they enjoyed or who stopped going to certain events or restaurants because there was nothing they could eat there. Well, cheer up. You don't need to follow a "diabetic diet" anymore.

Your body needs adequate amounts of six essential nutrients to function normally. Three of these—water, vitamins, and minerals—provide no energy and do not affect blood glucose levels. The other three—carbohydrate, protein, and fat—provide your body with the energy it needs to work. This energy is measured in calories. Any food that contains calories can cause your blood glucose levels to rise. For your body to properly use these energy calories, it needs insulin. Whenever you eat, your food is digested and broken down or converted into your body's primary fuel source, glucose. While all energy nutrients are broken down into glucose, carbohydrates have a more direct effect on blood glucose levels. Protein and fat have a slower, more indirect effect on those levels. Understanding this can help you predict how food will affect your glucose levels.

To be successful in diabetes self-care, you need to make personal food choices that are compatible with your blood glucose goals and your tastes. Since carbohydrates have the greatest direct effect on glucose levels, determining the amount of carbohydrates that your body can manage well is a cornerstone in your glucose management. It's simple, really. But before you begin, you should take a close look at your perceptions, preconceptions, and habits regarding food and eating; they can make eating much more complicated than need be. Adjusting them can allow you to enjoy the freedom that simplicity brings—and allow you to enjoy eating while you control your diabetes.

To gain a better understanding of how to use food choices to control your blood sugar levels, you must pay attention to how individual foods act in your body.

The first step is for you to eat absolutely normally. Have the foods you usually eat, in the amounts you normally have, as frequently as you usually have them. Check food labels to determine which foods contain carbohydrate, then keep a running tally of the total grams of carbohydrate you eat throughout the entire day. Take detailed, honest notes.

Along with taking these notes, you need to test your blood glucose levels. Testing allows you to see how well your insulin level matches your carbohydrate intake. No matter its source, insulin works with the food you eat. If you eat too much food for the insulin that is available, your glucose level will be too high; if you eat too little, your glucose level will be too low.

It is important to know that any food has the ability to make blood sugar levels rise, but different types of food as well as different amounts will result in different blood sugar levels. You may find that overeating makes blood sugar levels increase rapidly and stay too high. Overeating may not allow insulin to do its job properly. If you listen to your body's hunger cues and respect the feeling of fullness, your blood glucose will rise more slowly and peak at a lower level. Insulin, in turn, will be able to do its job and keep blood sugars at a healthy level. This type of balanced eating helps control diabetes and helps you feel better.

Eating a variety of foods will also help ensure that you get the nutrients you need—not just the carbohydrate, protein, and fat but also the vitamins and minerals that are essential to good health.

REMINDER

DIETARY CONTROL

Your body needs adequate amounts of six essential nutrients to function normally: water, vitamins, minerals, carbohydrates, protein, and fat. The last three provide your body with the energy it needs to work. This energy is measured in calories. Any food that contains calories can cause your blood glucose levels to rise. For your body to properly use these energy calories, it needs insulin. To be successful in diabetes self-care, you need to make personal food choices that are compatible with your blood glucose goals and your tastes.

STAYING ACTIVE

Activity is one of the three cornerstones in the treatment of diabetes, along with food and medication. Moving toward a more physically active life is generally inexpensive, convenient, and easy and usually produces great rewards in terms of blood glucose control (due to improved insulin sensitivity) and a general feeling of well-being.

Being active needs to be fun. Otherwise, you're much less likely to stick with an active lifestyle. So, choose your activities accordingly, then go out and play at least a little every day.

USING MEDICATIONS TO TREAT DIABETES

For many people who have type 2 diabetes, using food and activity to control blood glucose is not enough. For them, diabetes medications can be lifesavers—helping to lower blood glucose levels and stave off diabetes complications.

People with type 1 diabetes make very little, if any, insulin, so they are dependent on insulin injections. Insulin injections have become extremely safe and simple, and virtually pain-free. And, they remain the most natural and effective way to treat high blood sugar in these individuals.

On the other hand, individuals with type 2 diabetes may depend on pills to help lower blood glucose levels. But there are usually multiple problems that need to be addressed, and one pill just can't do it all. Problems include insulin resistance by the body's cells, oversecretion of glucose by the liver, insufficient insulin production by the pancreas, and alternated rates of food digestion. Sometimes a combination of medications is much more effective at lowering glucose levels than is a single medicine.

WEIGHING THE BENEFITS

You may realize (or your doctor has told you) that being overweight—especially carrying too much fat in your abdominal area—hampers diabetes control. For people with diabetes, the best path to weight loss is the same one that leads to getting well and staying well. There's no denying weight loss is beneficial for people with type 2 diabetes who are overweight. Even a weight loss of just 5 to 10 percent of your total body weight can bring impressive improvements to your health. Studies show that when a person who has recently been diagnosed with diabetes loses weight, blood glucose levels drop, blood pressure improves, and cholesterol levels return to a healthier range. Medications may be decreased or even stopped altogether.

Basically, changes that will help improve your glucose control include:

- **FILLING UP ON FIBER.** Foods high in fiber can help you feel fuller longer with fewer calories and without increasing blood sugar.

- **THINK SMALL.** Choose smaller, more reasonable portions on a smaller plate, and eat more slowly so you'll know it when your stomach is full.

- **CHECK THIRST.** Most people confuse feelings of thirst for hunger. Try reaching for a low-calorie beverage or water first before eating.

- **MAKE TRADES.** Choose foods that are lower in fat and light in calories instead of a higher calorie/fat dense food.

- **ADD MORE ACTIVITY.** The more you move, the more you'll lose.

TAKING COMMAND OF YOUR CARE

The right approach to diabetes treatment puts YOU in charge. Not your doctor. Not your spouse. YOU. You become the boss of your diabetes team, choosing the staff that best serves your needs, tracking your progress, and keeping your eyes on the ultimate goal—your health and well-being.

YOUR DIABETES TEAM

Surround yourself with knowledgeable, trustworthy, and expert advisors—your diabetes care team—who can help your get the information, advice, treatments, and support you need to manage your diabetes effectively. This team should include your doctor (possibly an endocrinologist who typically has the most experience and skill in diabetes care) and a registered dietitian nutritionist (RDN) who may also be certified as a diabetes educator (CDE) to teach people with diabetes how to manage the disease. Also onboard should be a pharmacist, dentist, mental-health professional, eye doctor, podiatrist, and cardiologist, as needed.

Your team will help you choose what, how much, and when to eat; help you become more physically active; assist with your medications; check your blood glucose; and teach you all they can about diabetes.

YOU'RE ON YOUR WAY

Once you feel comfortable with your meal and activity plan, checking your blood sugar, and managing your medication, you'll be able to enjoy the great taste of food without worries. Use the following recipes to get started on the path to a healthier lifestyle.

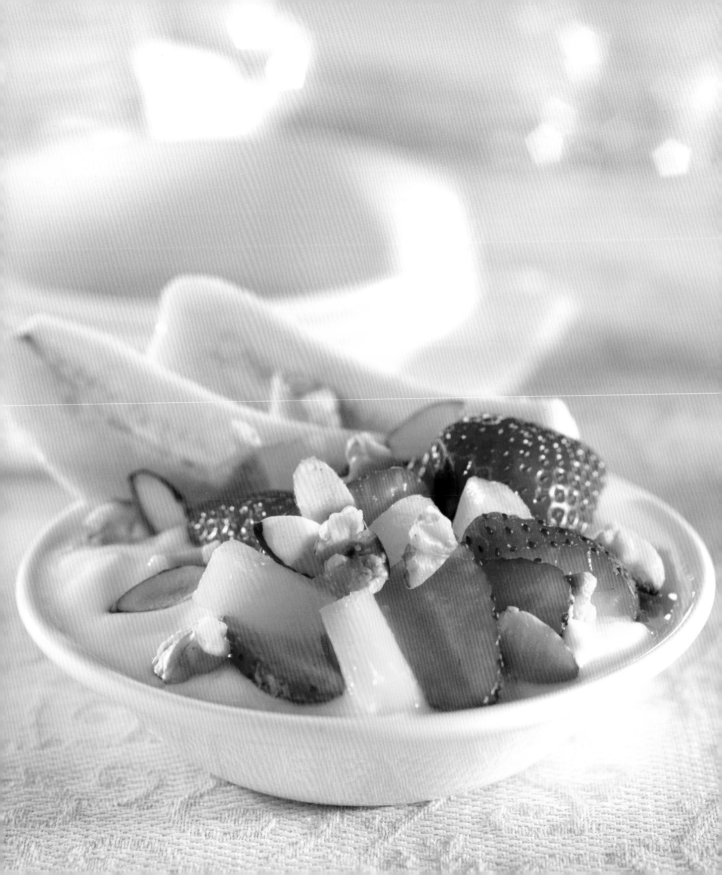

QUALITY BREAKFASTS

BANANA SPLIT BREAKFAST BOWL

MAKES 4 SERVINGS

1. Combine almonds and walnuts in small skillet; cook and stir over medium heat 2 minutes or until lightly browned. Immediately remove from skillet; cool completely.

2. Spoon yogurt into serving bowl. Layer with strawberries, bananas and pineapple; sprinkle with toasted almonds and walnuts.

NOTE: Recipes like this one can be made with fresh or frozen strawberries. Frozen fruits are economical, convenient and available year-round.

- $2\frac{1}{2}$ tablespoons sliced almonds
- $2\frac{1}{2}$ tablespoons chopped walnuts
- 3 cups vanilla nonfat yogurt
- $1\frac{1}{3}$ cups sliced fresh strawberries (about 12 medium)
- 2 bananas, sliced
- $\frac{1}{2}$ cup drained pineapple tidbits

Calories 268, **Total Fat** 5g, **Saturated Fat** 1g, **Cholesterol** 0mg, **Sodium** 112mg, **Carbohydrates** 50g, **Dietary Fiber** 5g, **Protein** 10g
Dietary Exchanges: 2 Fruit, 1 Milk, 1 Fat

OATMEAL WITH APPLES AND COTTAGE CHEESE

MAKES 2 SERVINGS

MICROWAVE DIRECTIONS

Combine first 7 ingredients in large microwave-safe bowl and stir. Cover with wet towel and microwave on HIGH 2 minutes; let stand 2 minutes. Add remaining ingredients, stir to combine and serve.

1/2 cup uncooked oats

1/2 cup diced apple

2/3 cup water

1/2 cup low-fat (1%) cottage cheese

3/4 teaspoon ground cinnamon

1 teaspoon vanilla

Dash salt (optional)

1/4 cup fat-free half-and-half

2 tablespoons chopped pecans or almonds

1 1/2 tablespoons sugar substitute*

This recipe was tested using sucralose-based sugar substitute.

Calories 205, **Total Fat** 7g, **Saturated Fat** 1g, **Cholesterol** 4mg, **Sodium** 275mg, **Carbohydrates** 25g, **Dietary Fiber** 4g, **Protein** 11g
Dietary Exchanges: 1 1/2 Bread/Starch, 1 Fat

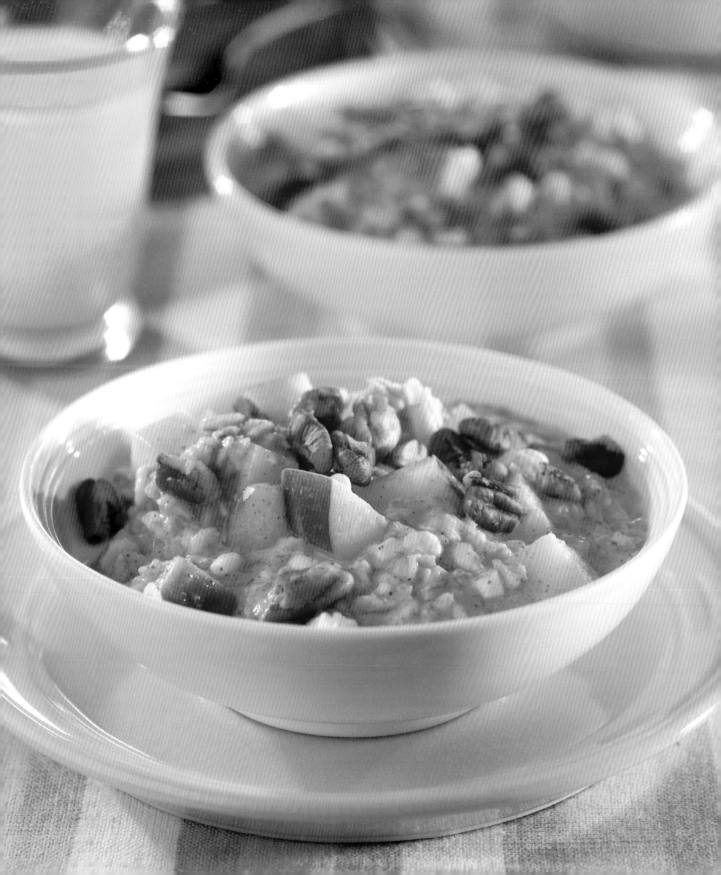

BREAKFAST TRAIL MIX

MAKES 4 SERVINGS (³/₄ CUP PER SERVING)

1. Heat large nonstick skillet over medium-high heat.

2. Combine all ingredients except salt in skillet; cook 3 minutes or until almonds are beginning to lightly brown. Stir frequently, separating bits of lemon peel while stirring. Remove from heat. Transfer to cookie sheet; spread in single layer. Sprinkle evenly with salt; cool completely.

3. Store cooled mixture in airtight container at room temperature.

2 cups high-fiber cereal*

¹/₂ cup slivered almonds

¹/₄ cup salted pumpkin seeds

¹/₄ cup dried apricots, chopped (about 10 halves)

1 tablespoon grated lemon peel

¹/₈ teaspoon salt

You may use oatmeal square cereal or high-protein, high-fiber breakfast cereal clusters.

Calories 255, **Total Fat** 12g, **Saturated Fat** 2g, **Cholesterol** 1mg, **Sodium** 240mg, **Carbohydrates** 26g, **Dietary Fiber** 6g, **Protein** 9g
Dietary Exchanges: 2 Bread/Starch, 2¹/₂ Fat

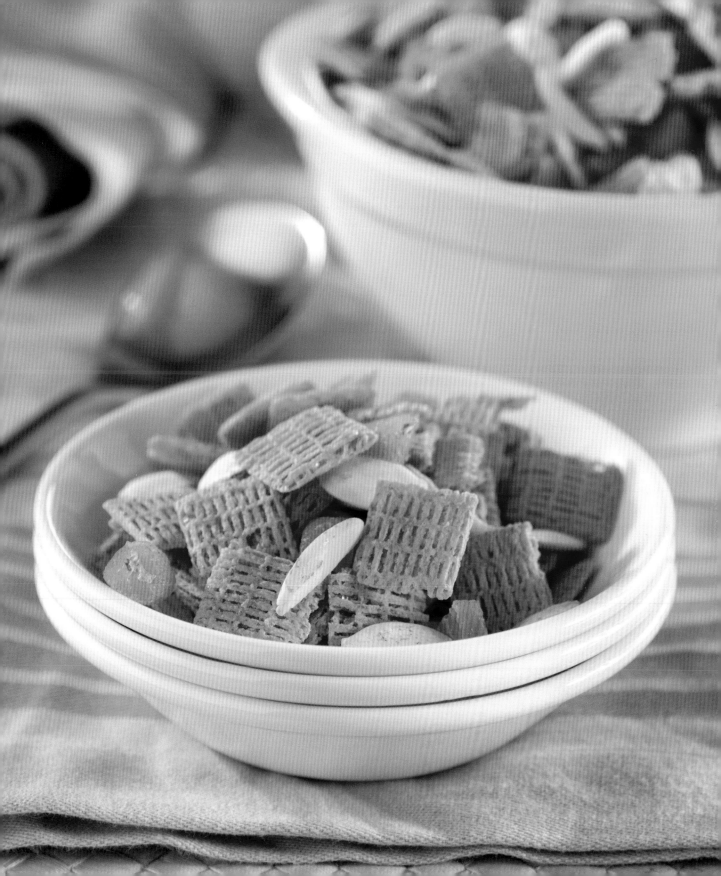

BREAKFAST COMFORT IN A CUP
MAKES 4 SERVINGS (1 CUP PER SERVING)

1. Spread 1 teaspoon margarine on each bread slice. Toast until lightly browned; cut into $1/2$-inch cubes.

2. Meanwhile, heat large skillet coated with nonstick cooking spray over medium heat. Add ham; cook 3 minutes or until beginning to lightly brown, stirring occasionally. Add egg substitute; tilt skillet to coat bottom, stirring occasionally until almost set. Fold in toast cubes, cheese, pepper and salt, if desired.

3. Spoon equal amounts in each of four cups, bowls or travel mugs.

NOTE: This breakfast will keep you going throughout the morning. You can even eat it on-the-go!

TIP: For a variation, you may substitute diced ham with turkey breakfast sausage links.

4 teaspoons reduced-fat margarine

4 slices reduced-calorie whole wheat bread, toasted

3 ounces 96% fat-free diced ham

1 cup cholesterol-free egg substitute

$1/4$ cup (1 ounce) reduced-fat sharp Cheddar cheese, grated

$1/4$ teaspoon black pepper

$1/8$ teaspoon salt (optional)

Calories 130, **Total Fat** 4g, **Saturated Fat** 2g, **Cholesterol** 16mg, **Sodium** 550mg, **Carbohydrates** 12g, **Dietary Fiber** 3g, **Protein** 13g
Dietary Exchanges: $1/2$ Bread/Starch, 2 Meat

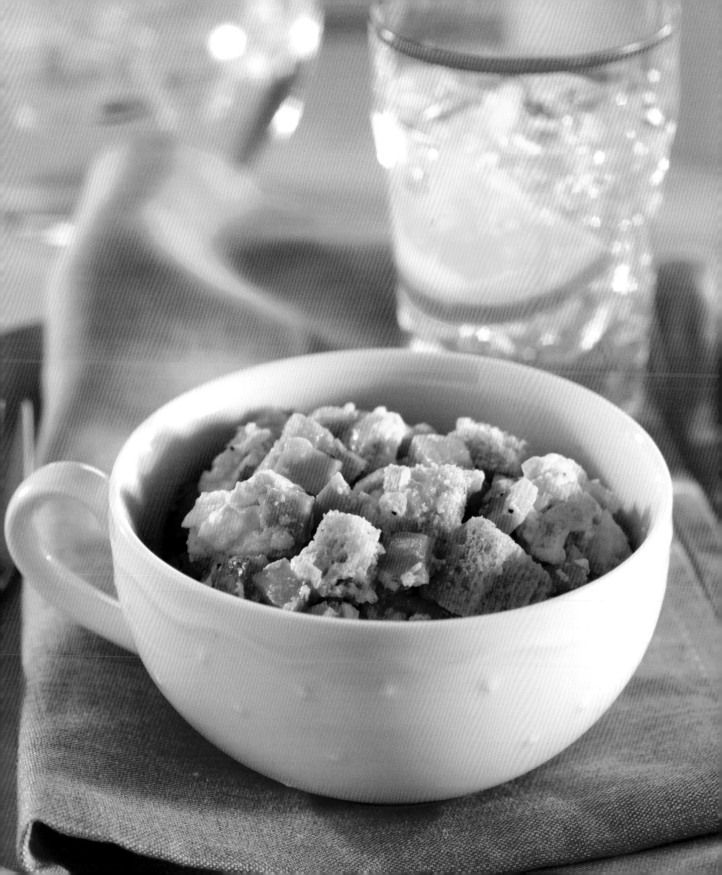

ASPARAGUS AND GREEN ONION OMELET WITH TORTILLA WEDGES

MAKES 2 SERVINGS

1. Preheat oven to 425°F. Place asparagus on baking sheet. Season with 1/8 teaspoon pepper; brush with oil. Roast 15 minutes, or until asparagus are golden brown and tender, shaking baking sheet occasionally. Remove and keep warm.

2. Beat egg whites until foamy in large bowl. Add remaining 1/8 teaspoon pepper, salt, chili powder, green onions and Parmesan cheese.

3. Coat large skillet with nonstick cooking spray. Pour in egg white mixture. Cook over medium-high heat until edges of omelet are firm and lightly browned. Lift omelet at edges to allow uncooked mixture to flow underneath. Continue cooking until egg whites are firm and dry. Cut omelet in half; arrange each half on plate. Serve with asparagus and tortilla wedges.

8 ounces small asparagus spears, ends cut off

1/4 teaspoon black pepper, divided

1 teaspoon olive oil

5 large egg whites

1/8 teaspoon salt

1/16 teaspoon chipotle chili powder

2 tablespoons chopped green onions

1/4 cup shredded Parmesan cheese

1 (8-inch) whole wheat tortilla, heated and cut into wedges*

Or, you may substitute with 1 whole wheat pita bread round, cut in half.

Calories 152, **Total Fat** 4g, **Saturated Fat** 1g, **Cholesterol** 1mg, **Sodium** 449mg, **Carbohydrates** 14g, **Dietary Fiber** 2g, **Protein** 15g
Dietary Exchanges: 1 Bread/Starch, 2 Meat

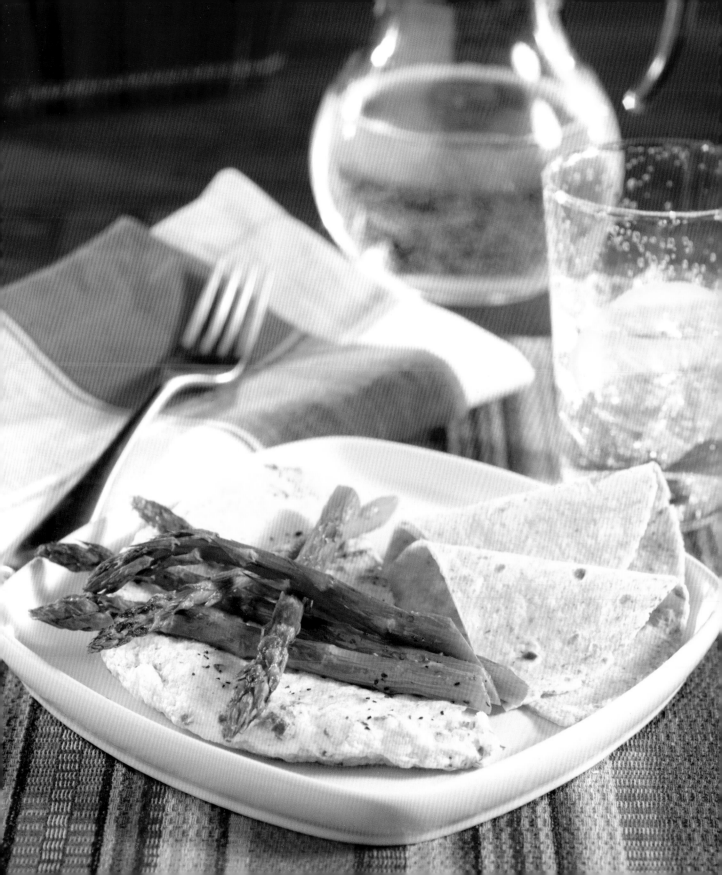

MEDITERRANEAN SCRAMBLE PITAS

MAKES 4 SERVINGS

1. Heat 1 teaspoon oil in large nonstick skillet over medium-high heat. Add zucchini and bell peppers; cook 4 minutes or until crisp-tender. Add tomatoes and rosemary; cook 2 minutes, stirring frequently. Stir in olives and parsley. Place in medium bowl. Cover to keep warm.

2. Wipe out skillet with paper towel. Add remaining 1 teaspoon oil and heat over medium heat. Cook egg substitute until set, lifting edges to allow uncooked portion to flow underneath.

3. Fill each warmed pita half with equal amounts of eggs and feta. Top with vegetable mixture and remaining feta.

2 teaspoons canola oil, divided

1 cup sliced zucchini and/or yellow squash

1 cup diced green bell peppers

1 cup grape tomatoes, quartered

$1/4$ teaspoon dried rosemary

12 small stuffed green olives, quartered

$1/4$ cup finely chopped fresh Italian parsley

1 cup cholesterol-free egg substitute

2 multigrain pita bread rounds, halved and warmed

1 ounce reduced-fat feta cheese, crumbled

Calories 199, **Total Fat** 7g, **Saturated Fat** 1g, **Cholesterol** 2mg, **Sodium** 554mg, **Carbohydrates** 26g, **Dietary Fiber** 6g, **Protein** 12g
Dietary Exchanges: 1 Bread/Starch, 1 Meat

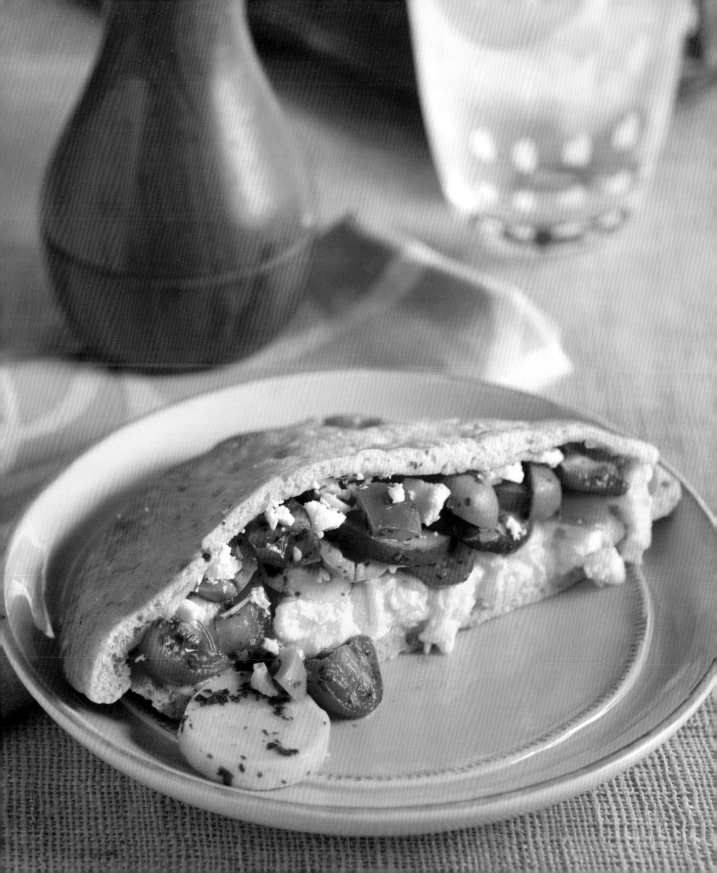

BREAKFAST QUESADILLAS

MAKES 4 SERVINGS

1. Whisk egg substitute and milk in small bowl. Heat 2 teaspoons oil in large skillet over medium heat. Cook eggs until set, lifting edges to allow uncooked portion to flow underneath. Remove from skillet. Wipe out skillet with paper towel.

2. Spread 1 tablespoon chiles on half of each tortilla. Top each with eggs, cheese and cilantro; sprinkle evenly with pepperoni. Fold tortillas in half.

3. Heat remaining 2 teaspoons oil in skillet. Cook quesadillas in two batches 3 minutes per side or until cheese is melted.

1 cup cholesterol-free egg substitute

2 tablespoons fat-free (skim) milk

4 teaspoons canola oil, divided

1 can (4 ounces) chopped mild green chiles

8 soft corn tortillas

1/2 cup (2 ounces) shredded reduced-fat sharp Cheddar cheese

1/4 cup chopped fresh cilantro

1 ounce turkey pepperoni slices, quartered

Calories 246, **Total Fat** 10g, **Saturated Fat** 3g, **Cholesterol** 19mg, **Sodium** 490mg, **Carbohydrates** 25g, **Dietary Fiber** 3g, **Protein** 15g
Dietary Exchanges: 1½ Bread/Starch, 1½ Meat, 1 Fat

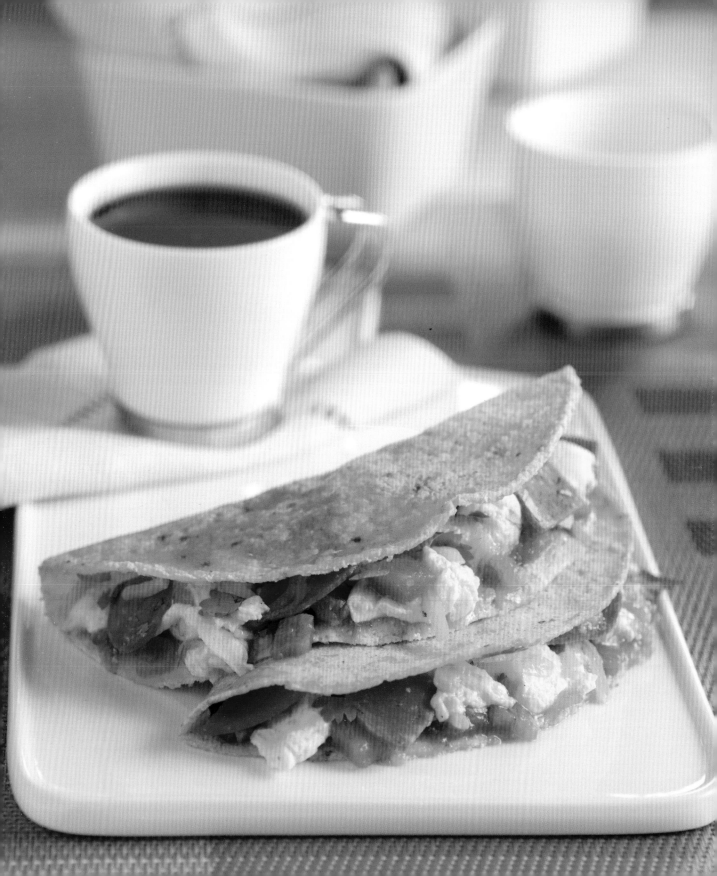

WHOLE-WHEAT PUMPKIN MUFFINS

MAKES 12 MUFFINS

1. Preheat oven to 350°F. Spray 12 standard (2½-inch) muffin cups with nonstick cooking spray.

2. Combine flour, sugar, salt, allspice, nutmeg, baking powder and baking soda in large bowl; mix well. Stir in pumpkin, oil, honey and apple juice concentrate until well blended. Stir in walnuts and raisins. Spoon evenly into prepared muffin cups.

3. Bake 12 to 15 minutes or until toothpick inserted into centers comes out clean. Remove to wire rack; cool completely.

1½ cups whole wheat flour

¼ cup sugar

1 teaspoon salt

1 teaspoon ground allspice

1 teaspoon ground nutmeg

¾ teaspoon baking powder

½ teaspoon baking soda

¾ cup canned pumpkin

½ cup canola oil

½ cup honey

½ cup frozen apple juice concentrate, thawed

½ cup chopped walnuts

½ cup golden raisins

Calories 268, **Total Fat** 12g, **Saturated Fat** 1g, **Cholesterol** 0mg, **Sodium** 283mg, **Carbohydrates** 39g, **Dietary Fiber** 3g, **Protein** 3g
Dietary Exchanges: 2½ Bread/Starch, 2 Fat

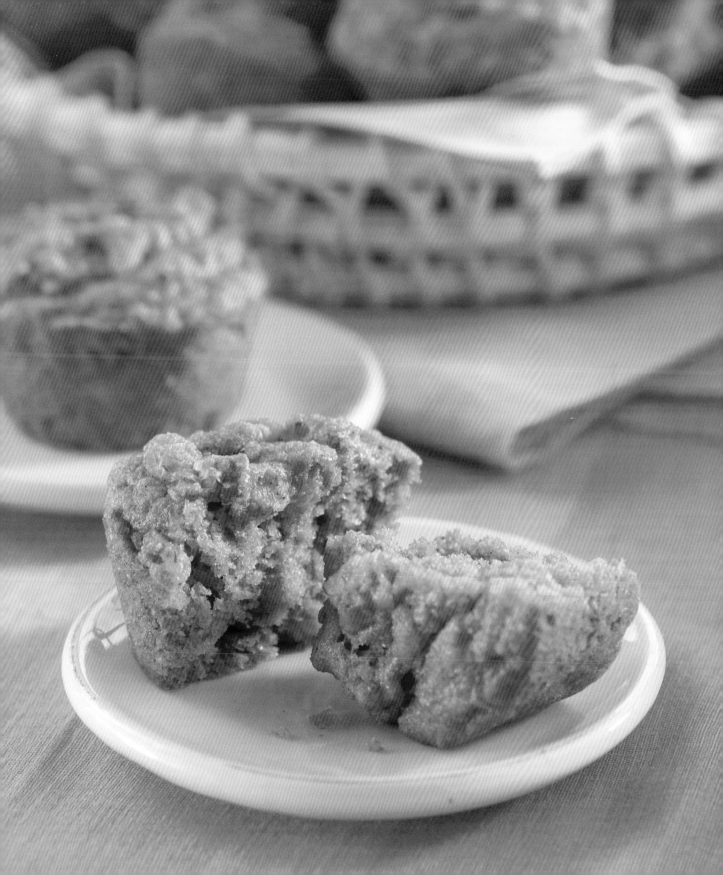

FRUIT KABOBS WITH RASPBERRY YOGURT DIP

MAKES 6 SERVINGS

1. Stir yogurt and fruit spread in small bowl until well blended.

2. Thread fruit alternately onto six 12-inch skewers. Serve with yogurt dip.

½ cup plain nonfat yogurt

¼ cup no-sugar-added raspberry fruit spread

1 pint fresh strawberries

2 cups cubed honeydew melon (1-inch cubes)

2 cups cubed cantaloupe (1-inch cubes)

1 can (8 ounces) pineapple chunks in juice, drained

Calories 108, **Total Fat** 1g, **Saturated Fat** 1g, **Cholesterol** 1mg, **Sodium** 52mg, **Carbohydrates** 25g, **Dietary Fiber** 2g, **Protein** 2g
Dietary Exchanges: 2 Fruit

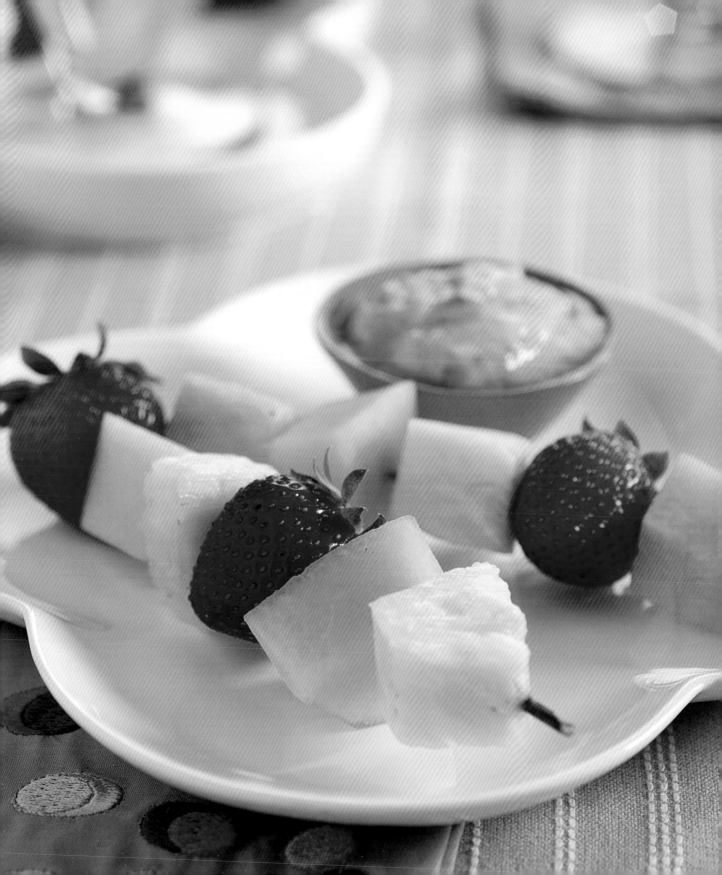

HAM & EGG BREAKFAST PANINI

MAKES 2 SANDWICHES

1. Spray small skillet with nonstick cooking spray; heat over medium heat. Add bell pepper and green onion; cook and stir 4 minutes or until crisp-tender. Stir in ham.

2. Whisk egg substitute and black pepper in small bowl until well blended. Pour egg mixture into skillet; cook 2 minutes or until egg mixture is almost set, stirring occasionally.

3. Heat grill pan or medium skillet over medium heat. Spray one side of each bread slice with cooking spray; turn bread over. Top 2 bread slices with 1 cheese slice and half of egg mixture. Top with remaining bread slices.

4. Grill 2 minutes per side, pressing down lightly with spatula until toasted. (Cover pan with lid during last 2 minutes of cooking to melt cheese, if desired.) Serve immediately.

1/4 cup chopped green or red bell pepper

2 tablespoons sliced green onion

1 slice (1 ounce) reduced-fat smoked deli ham, chopped

1/2 cup cholesterol-free egg substitute

Black pepper

4 slices multigrain or whole grain bread

2 slices (3/4-ounce each) reduced-fat Cheddar or Swiss cheese

Calories 271, **Total Fat** 5g, **Saturated Fat** 1g, **Cholesterol** 9mg, **Sodium** 577mg, **Carbohydrates** 30g, **Dietary Fiber** 6g, **Protein** 24g
Dietary Exchanges: 2 Bread/Starch, 2 Meat

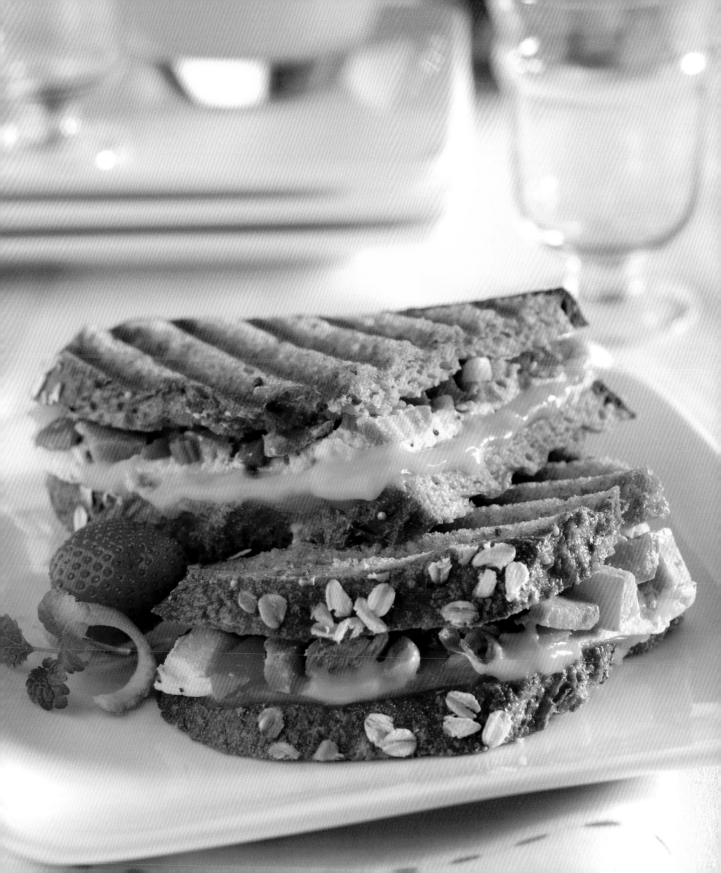

COTTAGE CHEESE BREAKFAST PARFAITS

MAKES 4 SERVINGS

1. Combine cantaloupe, honeydew, grapes and strawberries in medium bowl.

2. Layer one third of cottage cheese in four short wide drinking glasses or wide wine glasses; top with half of fruit and half of almonds. Repeat layering with one third of cottage cheese, remaining fruit, remaining cottage cheese and remaining almonds. Sprinkle with nutmeg, if desired.

NOTE: This recipe is best if served immediately. Making the parfaits too far in advanced will cause the melon to weep into the cottage cheese.

$1/2$ cup $1/2$-inch diced cantaloupe cubes

$1/2$ cup $1/2$-inch diced honeydew cubes

1 cup halved green or red seedless grapes

1 cup sliced fresh strawberries

1 container (16 ounces) low-fat (1%) cottage cheese

$1/4$ cup toasted sliced almonds

Ground nutmeg (optional)

Calories 167, **Total Fat** 4g, **Saturated Fat** 1g, **Cholesterol** 5mg, **Sodium** 468mg, **Carbohydrates** 17g, **Dietary Fiber** 2g, **Protein** 16g
Dietary Exchanges: 2 Meat, 1 Fruit

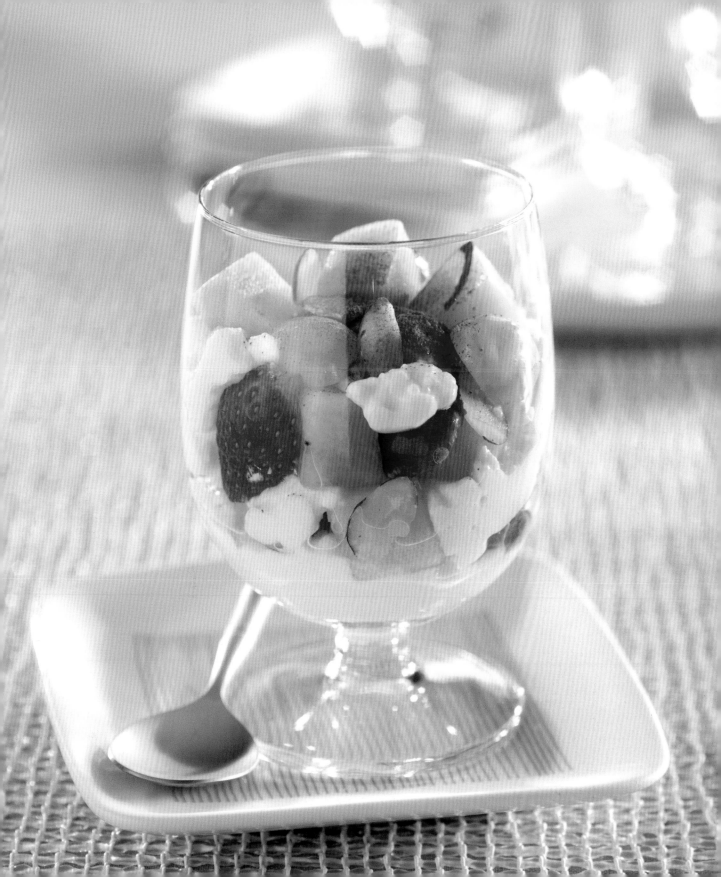

HAM AND VEGETABLE OMELET

MAKES 4 SERVINGS

1. Spray large nonstick skillet with nonstick cooking spray; heat over medium-high heat. Add ham, onion, bell peppers and garlic; cook and stir 5 minutes or until vegetables are crisp-tender. Transfer mixture to large bowl.

2. Wipe out skillet with paper towels; spray with cooking spray. Heat over medium-high heat. Pour egg substitute into skillet; sprinkle with black pepper. Cook 2 minutes or until bottom is set, lifting edge of egg with spatula to allow uncooked portion to flow underneath. Reduce heat to medium-low; cover and cook 4 minutes or until top is set.

3. Gently slide omelet onto large serving plate; spoon ham mixture down center. Sprinkle with 1/4 cup cheese. Carefully fold two sides of omelet over ham mixture; sprinkle with remaining 1/4 cup cheese and tomato. Cut into four wedges; serve immediately with hot pepper sauce, if desired.

2 ounces (about 1/2 cup) diced 95% fat-free ham

1 small onion, diced

1/2 medium green bell pepper, diced

1/2 medium red bell pepper, diced

2 cloves garlic, minced

1 1/2 cups cholesterol-free egg substitute

1/8 teaspoon black pepper

1/2 cup (2 ounces) shredded reduced-fat Colby cheese, divided

1 medium tomato, chopped

Hot pepper sauce (optional)

Calories 126, **Total Fat** 4g, **Saturated Fat** 2g, **Cholesterol** 17mg, **Sodium** 443mg, **Carbohydrates** 8g, **Dietary Fiber** 1g, **Protein** 16g
Dietary Exchanges: 2 Meat, 1 Vegetable

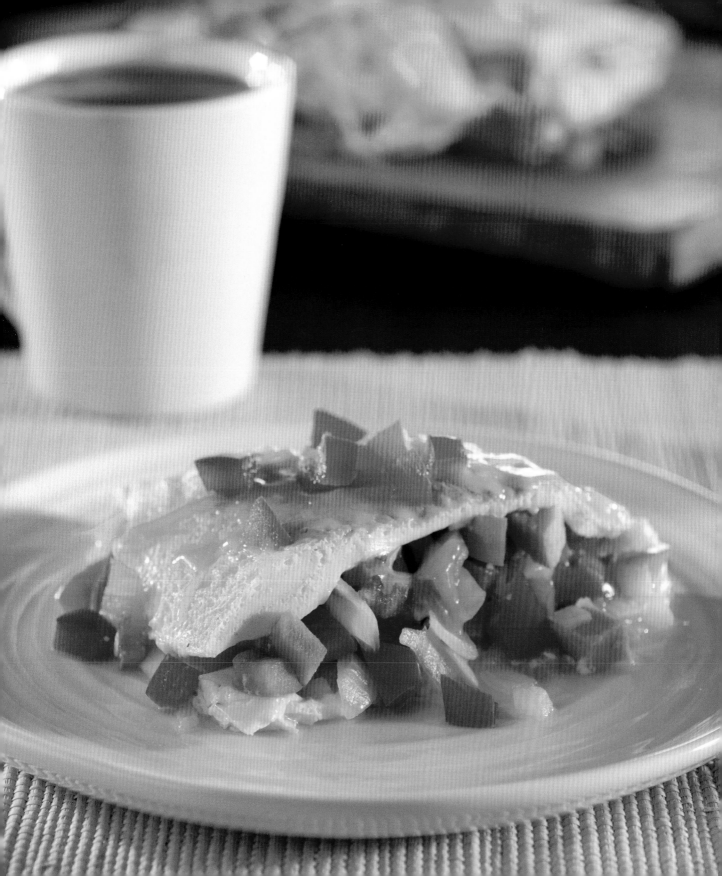

VANILLA MULTIGRAIN WAFFLES

MAKES 4 WAFFLES

1. Combine buttermilk and oats in large bowl; let stand 10 minutes. Spray waffle maker with nonstick cooking spray; preheat according to manufacturer's directions.

2. Combine all-purpose flour, whole wheat flour, baking powder, baking soda and salt in medium bowl; mix well.

3. Whisk egg, brown sugar, oil and vanilla in small bowl until smooth and well blended. Stir into oat mixture. Add flour mixture; stir until smooth and well blended.

4. Pour $2/3$ cup batter into waffle maker; cook about 5 minutes or until steam stops escaping from around edges and waffle is golden brown. Repeat with remaining batter. Serve with maple syrup, if desired.

1 cup low-fat buttermilk

¼ cup steel cut oats

⅓ cup all-purpose flour

⅓ cup whole wheat flour

1 teaspoon baking powder

½ teaspoon baking soda

¼ teaspoon salt

1 egg

2 tablespoons packed brown sugar

1 tablespoon vegetable oil

1 teaspoon vanilla

Sugar-free maple syrup (optional)

Calories 212, **Total Fat** 6g, **Saturated Fat** 1g, **Cholesterol** 49mg, **Sodium** 509mg, **Carbohydrates** 32g, **Dietary Fiber** 2g, **Protein** 7g
Dietary Exchanges: 2 Bread/Starch, 1 Fat

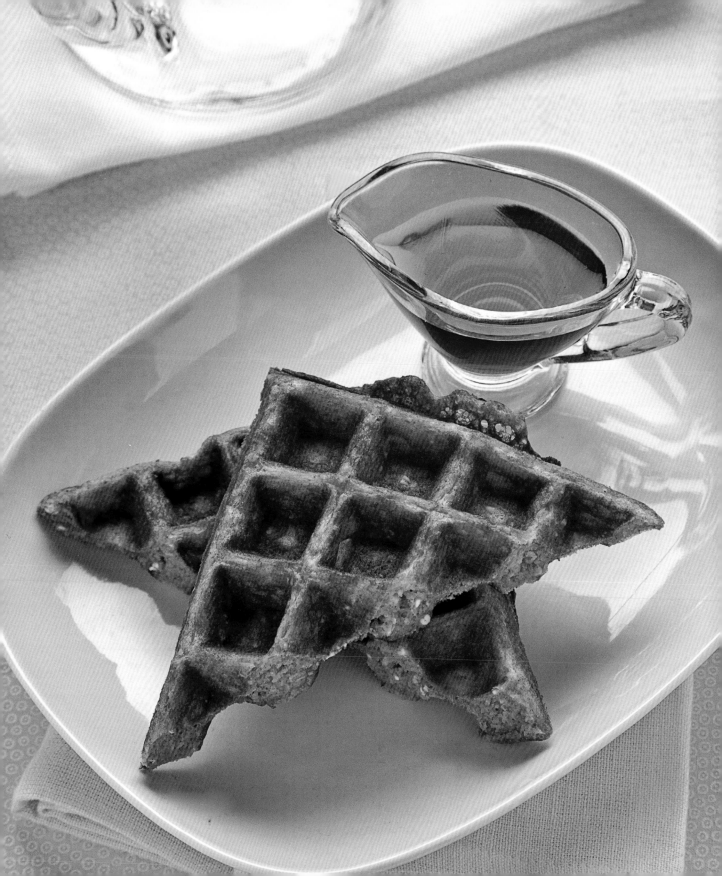

FRUITED GRANOLA

MAKES ABOUT 20 SERVINGS

1. Preheat oven to 325°F.

2. Spread oats and almonds in single layer in 13×9-inch baking pan. Bake 15 minutes or until lightly toasted, stirring frequently.

3. Combine honey, wheat germ, butter and cinnamon in large bowl until well blended. Add oats and almonds; toss to coat completely. Spread mixture in single layer in baking pan. Bake 20 minutes or until golden brown. Cool completely in pan on wire rack. Break mixture into chunks.

4. Combine oat chunks, cereal, blueberries, cranberries and banana chips in large bowl. Store in airtight container at room temperature up to 2 weeks.

TIP: Prepare this granola on the weekend and you'll have a scrumptious snack or breakfast treat on hand for the rest of the week!

3 cups quick-cooking oats

1 cup sliced almonds

1 cup honey

$1/2$ cup wheat germ or honey wheat germ

3 tablespoons butter or margarine, melted

1 teaspoon ground cinnamon

3 cups whole grain cereal flakes

$1/2$ cup dried blueberries or golden raisins

$1/2$ cup dried cranberries or cherries

$1/2$ cup dried banana chips or chopped pitted dates

Calories 210, **Total Fat** 7g, **Saturated Fat** 2g, **Cholesterol** 5mg, **Sodium** 58mg, **Carbohydrates** 36g, **Dietary Fiber** 4g, **Protein** 5g
Dietary Exchanges: 2 Bread/Starch, 1½ Fat

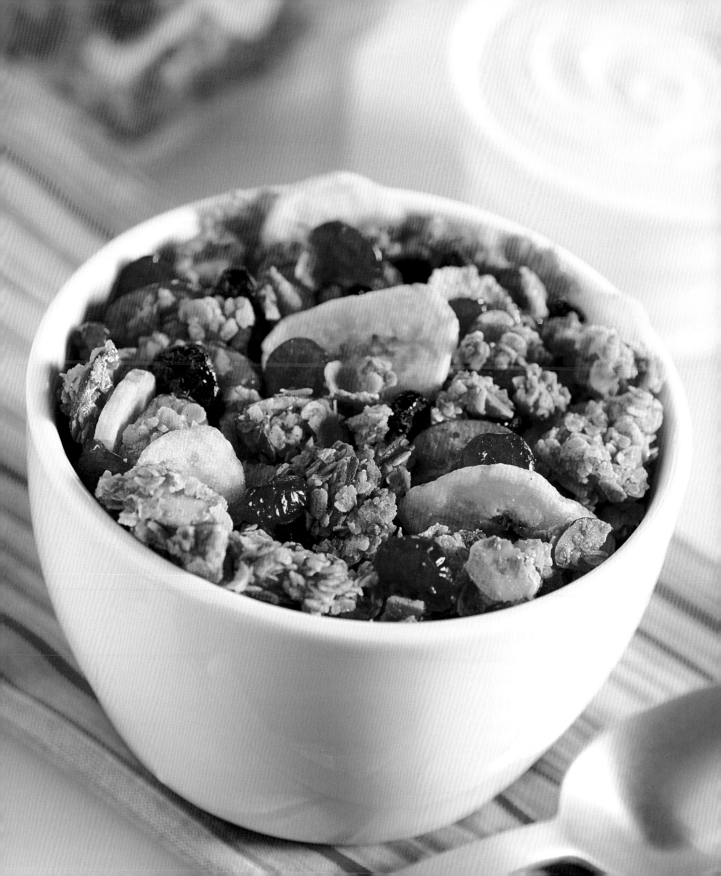

BREAKFAST PIZZA MARGHERITA

MAKES 6 SERVINGS

1. Preheat oven to 450°F. Place pizza crust on 12-inch pizza pan. Bake 6 to 8 minutes or until heated through.

2. Meanwhile, coat large skillet with nonstick cooking spray. Cook bacon over medium-high heat until crisp. Remove from skillet to paper towels; cool. Crumble bacon.

3. Combine egg substitute, milk, $1/2$ tablespoon basil and pepper in medium bowl. Coat same skillet with cooking spray. Add egg substitute mixture. Cook over medium heat until mixture begins to set around edges. Gently stir eggs, allowing uncooked portions to flow underneath. Repeat stirring of egg mixture every 1 to 2 minutes or until eggs are just set. Remove from heat.

4. Arrange tomato slices on warmed pizza crust. Spoon scrambled eggs over tomatoes. Sprinkle with bacon. Top with cheeses. Bake 1 minute or until cheese is melted. Sprinkle with remaining 1 tablespoon basil. Cut into six wedges. Serve immediately.

- 1 (12-inch) prepared pizza crust
- 3 slices 95% fat-free turkey bacon
- 2 cups cholesterol-free egg substitute
- $1/2$ cup fat-free (skim) milk
- $1^{1}/_{2}$ tablespoons chopped fresh basil, divided
- $1/8$ teaspoon black pepper
- 2 plum tomatoes, thinly sliced
- $1/2$ cup (2 ounces) shredded reduced-fat mozzarella cheese
- $1/4$ cup (1 ounce) shredded reduced-fat Cheddar cheese

Calories 311, **Total Fat** 9g, **Saturated Fat** 2g, **Cholesterol** 11mg, **Sodium** 675mg, **Carbohydrates** 35g, **Dietary Fiber** 2g, **Protein** 21g
Dietary Exchanges: 2 Bread/Starch, 2 Meat, $1/2$ Vegetable, $1^{1}/_{2}$ Fat

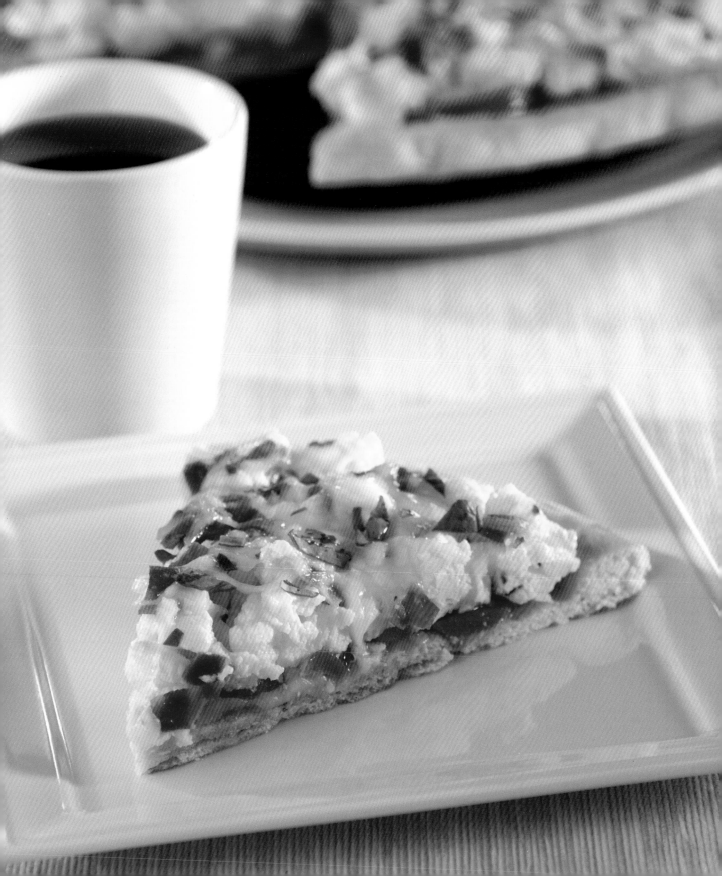

MORNING SANDWICHES

MAKES 6 SERVINGS

1. Preheat oven to 425°F. Spray 13×9-inch baking pan with nonstick cooking spray.

2. Melt butter in small nonstick saucepan over medium heat. Add oats and almonds; cook and stir 3 minutes. Remove from heat; let cool.

3. Place oat mixture, flour, apple, carrots, egg substitute, prunes, milk, sugar substitute, baking powder, cinnamon, baking soda and nutmeg in food processor; pulse until combined. Press dough evenly into prepared pan.

4. Bake 20 minutes. Cool 15 minutes in pan on wire rack.

5. Cut into 12 pieces. Spread six pieces with peanut butter; spread remaining six pieces with raspberry preserves. Press pieces together to form sandwiches.

1 tablespoon butter or vegetable oil

2 ounces (³⁄₄ cup) quick oats

¼ cup sliced almonds

1 cup whole wheat flour

1 cup peeled and grated apple

1 cup shredded carrots

⅓ cup cholesterol-free egg substitute

¼ cup pitted and chopped prunes

¼ cup fat-free (skim) milk

2 tablespoons sugar substitute

½ teaspoon baking powder

½ teaspoon ground cinnamon

¼ teaspoon baking soda

¼ teaspoon ground nutmeg

6 teaspoons reduced-fat peanut butter

6 teaspoons sugar-free raspberry preserves

Calories 272, **Total Fat** 11g, **Saturated Fat** 2g, **Cholesterol** 6mg, **Sodium** 215mg, **Carbohydrates** 36g, **Dietary Fiber** 7g, **Protein** 10g
Dietary Exchanges: 2 Bread/Starch, ½ Fruit, 2 Fat

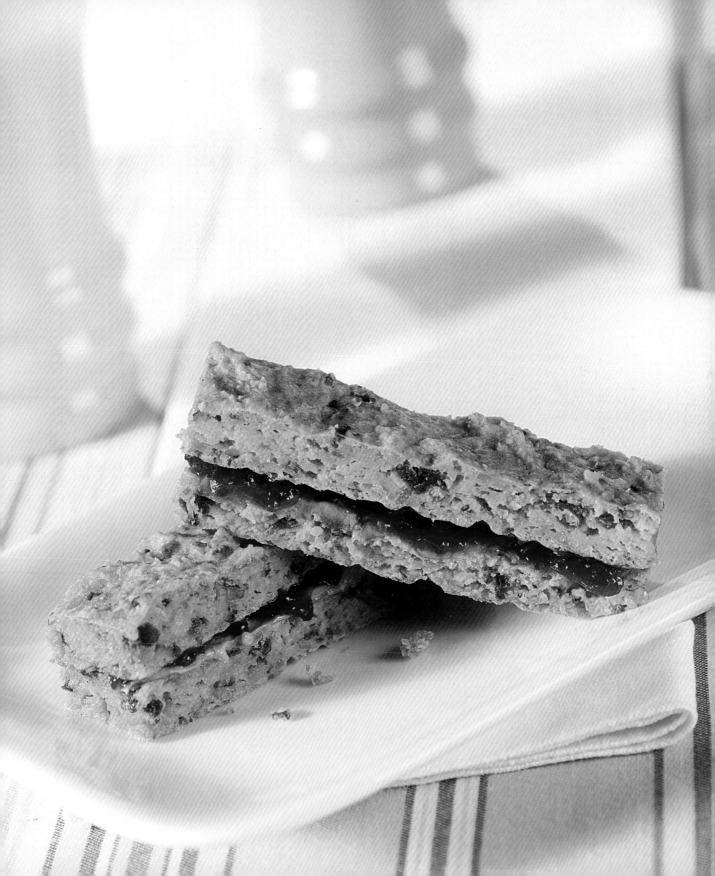

GREEN PEPPER SAUSAGE GRITS

MAKES 4 SERVINGS (1 CUP PER SERVING)

1. Bring 2 cups water to a boil in medium saucepan over high heat. Gradually stir in grits; reduce heat. Cover and simmer 6 minutes or until thickened, stirring occasionally. Stir in $1/8$ teaspoon salt. Set aside.

2. Meanwhile, spray large skillet with nonstick cooking spray; heat over medium-high heat. Add sausage; cook until browned, stirring to break up meat. Remove to plate.

3. Heat oil in same skillet over medium-high heat. Add bell pepper; cook and stir 3 minutes. Add tomatoes and garlic; cook 3 minutes or until softened. Stir in remaining $1/4$ cup water until well blended. Remove from heat.

4. Stir sausage and any accumulated juices, green onions, ground red pepper and remaining $1/8$ teaspoon salt into skillet.

5. Divide grits among four serving plates. Top with sausage mixture and parsley.

$2^1/4$ cups water, divided

$1/2$ cup quick-cooking grits

$1/4$ teaspoon salt, divided

6 ounces fully cooked turkey breakfast sausage links

2 teaspoons extra virgin olive oil

1 cup diced green bell pepper

1 cup grape tomatoes, quartered

2 cloves garlic, minced

$1/4$ cup finely chopped green onions

$1/8$ teaspoon ground red pepper

2 tablespoons chopped fresh parsley

Calories 210, **Total Fat** 10g, **Saturated Fat** 3g, **Cholesterol** 26mg, **Sodium** 545mg, **Carbohydrates** 21g, **Dietary Fiber** 2g, **Protein** 9g
Dietary Exchanges: 1 Bread/Starch, 1 Meat, 1 Vegetable, $1/2$ Fat

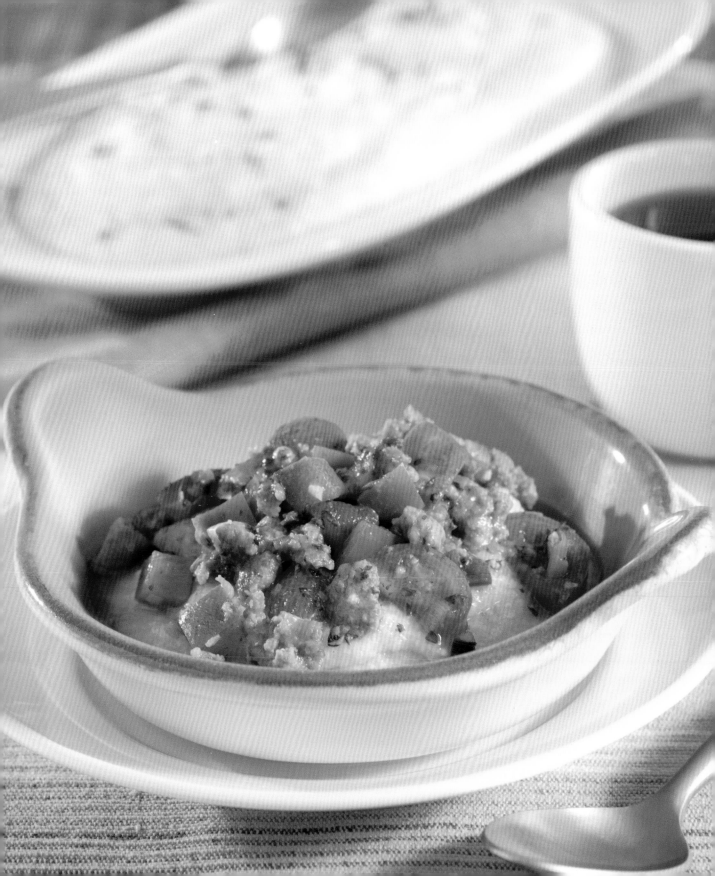

WHOLE-GRAIN CEREAL BARS

MAKES 24 BARS

1. Grease 13×19-inch baking pan.

2. Place cereal in large resealable food storage bag; seal bag. Using rolling pin, lightly roll over bag until cereals are crumbled.

3. Combine marshmallows and butter in large saucepan over medium-low heat; cook and stir until marshmallows are melted and mixture is smooth. Remove from heat.

4. Stir in cereal until well blended. Using waxed paper, press cereal mixture evenly into prepared pan. Sprinkle with oats. Let stand until firm. Cut into bars.

5 to 6 cups assorted whole grain cereals

1 package (10 ounces) large marshmallows

1/4 cup (1/2 stick) butter

1/4 cup old-fashioned oats

Calories 88, **Total Fat** 2g, **Saturated Fat** 1g, **Cholesterol** 5mg, **Sodium** 76mg, **Carbohydrates** 17g, **Dietary Fiber** 1g, **Protein** 1g
Dietary Exchanges: 1 Bread/Starch, 1/2 Fat

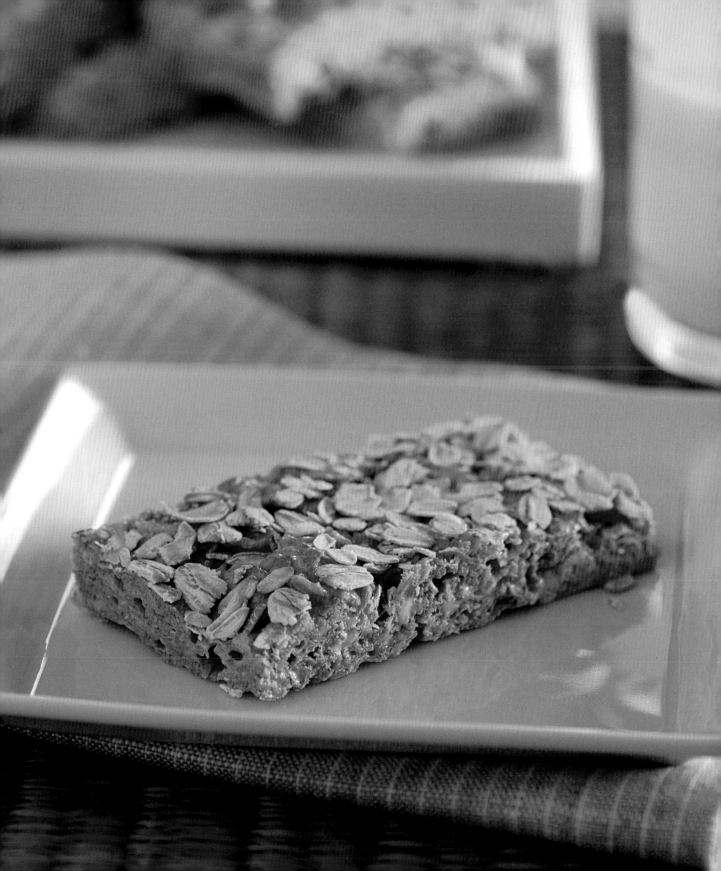

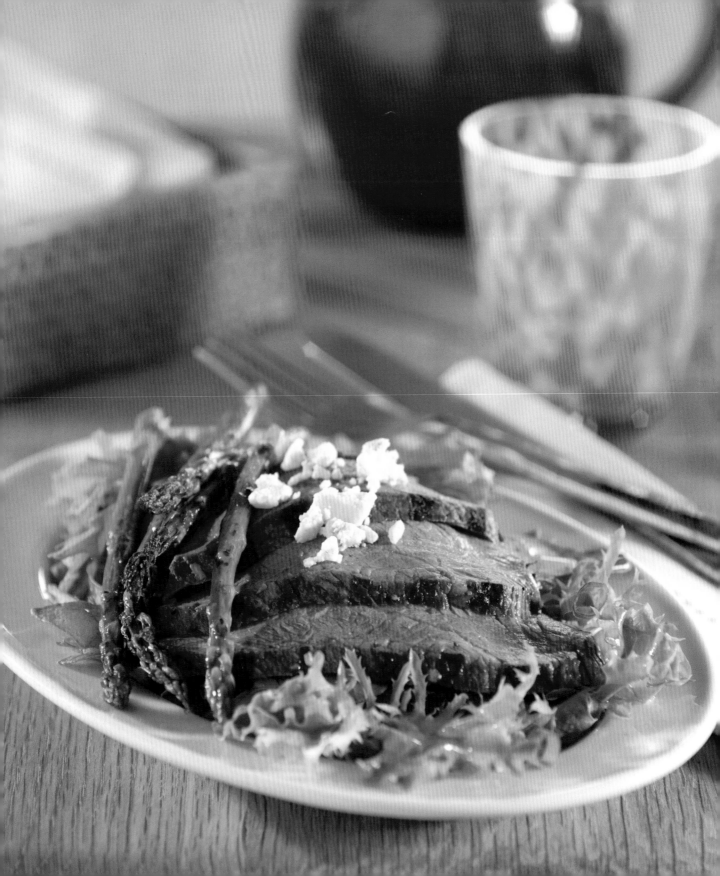

PLEASING LUNCHES

GRILLED STEAK AND ASPARAGUS SALAD

MAKES 4 SERVINGS

1. Prepare grill for direct cooking. Season steak with seasoning blend. Grill steak, covered, over medium heat about 8 to 10 minutes, turning once, until steak is still pink in center. Remove from grill. Cover loosely with foil to keep warm.

2. Place asparagus in grill basket; drizzle with oil and roll to coat. Grill over medium heat 3 to 5 minutes or until crisp-tender, shaking basket once or twice. Remove from grill.

3. Meanwhile, toss salad greens, green onions and vinaigrette in large bowl. Divide salad among four plates. Thinly slice steak across the grain. Divide among salad plates. Top each salad with asparagus and sprinkle with blue cheese.

1 boneless top sirloin steak (10 ounces and about 1-inch thick), trimmed of visible fat

1 teaspoon salt-free garlic-herb seasoning blend

1 pound fresh asparagus, trimmed

1 teaspoon canola oil

6 cups spring salad greens

1/2 cup chopped green onions

1/4 cup light champagne vinaigrette or other light vinaigrette

4 teaspoons crumbled blue cheese

Calories 189, **Total Fat** 8g, **Saturated Fat** 2g, **Cholesterol** 40mg, **Sodium** 198mg, **Carbohydrates** 10g, **Dietary Fiber** 3g, **Protein** 20g
Dietary Exchanges: 2 Meat, 2 Vegetable, 1/2 Fat

SHRIMP, FETA AND TOMATO SALAD

MAKES 4 SERVINGS

Combine shrimp, tomatoes, basil, oil, vinegar and pepper in medium bowl; mix well. Serve over lettuce and top with cheese.

- 8 ounces cooked medium shrimp, peeled and deveined (with tails on)
- 1 pint (2 cups) cherry tomatoes, halved (or whole small yellow pear tomatoes)
- 1/4 cup chopped or thinly sliced fresh basil
- 1 tablespoon olive oil
- 1 tablespoon white wine vinegar
- 1/4 teaspoon freshly ground black pepper
- 8 large Boston lettuce leaves
- 1/2 cup crumbled reduced-fat feta cheese

Calories 137, **Total Fat** 6g, **Saturated Fat** 2g, **Cholesterol** 100mg, **Sodium** 337mg, **Carbohydrates** 4g, **Dietary Fiber** 1g, **Protein** 16g
Dietary Exchanges: 2 Meat, 1 Vegetable

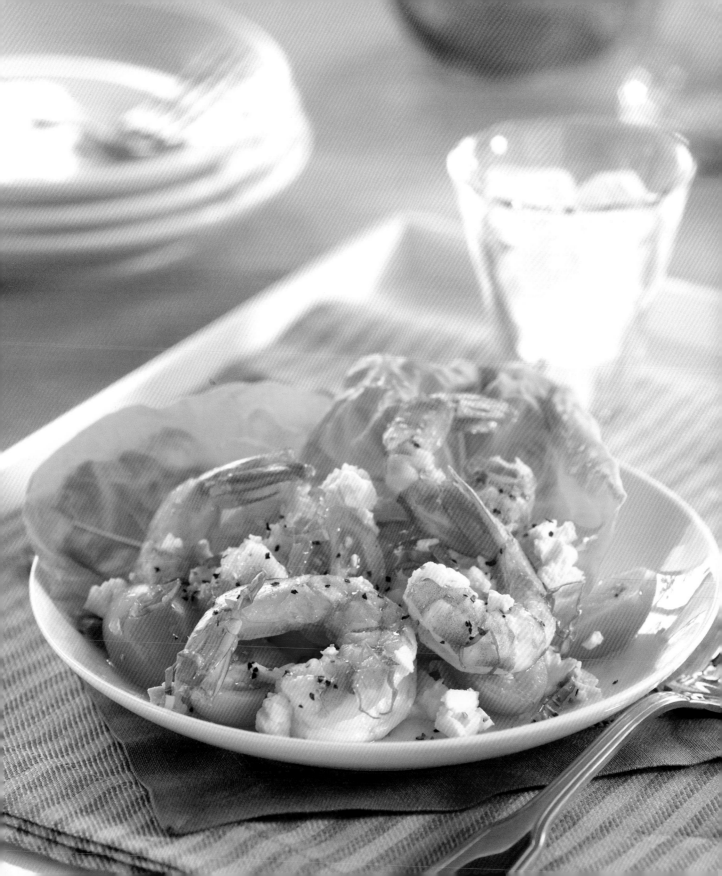

GARLIC BREAD AND SALMON SALAD

MAKES 4 SERVINGS (1 CUP PER SERVING)

1. Preheat broiler. Set rack 3 to 4 inches from heat. Rub one side of each bread slice with garlic. Discard garlic. Set bread, garlic side up, on broiler rack. Broil 20 to 30 seconds or until lightly browned; watch carefully and remove when done to avoid burning.

2. Set bread aside. When cool enough to handle, cut into 1-inch pieces.

3. Combine salmon, green onions and tomatoes in large serving bowl. Combine oil, vinegar, tomato juice, salt and pepper in cup. Pour over salmon mixture. Add garlic bread cubes and toss again. Sprinkle with basil.

2 slices day-old light whole wheat bread

1 clove garlic, cut in half

$7\frac{1}{2}$ ounces canned, pouch or cooked salmon, flaked

$\frac{1}{2}$ cup chopped green onions, green parts only

1 cup cherry or grape tomatoes, halved

1 teaspoon olive oil

5 teaspoons white wine vinegar

1 tablespoon tomato juice

$\frac{1}{4}$ teaspoon salt

$\frac{1}{4}$ teaspoon black pepper

2 tablespoons minced fresh basil

Calories 123, **Total Fat** 4g, **Saturated Fat** 1g, **Cholesterol** 44mg, **Sodium** 430mg, **Carbohydrates** 8g, **Dietary Fiber** 2g, **Protein** 15g
Dietary Exchanges: $\frac{1}{2}$ Bread/Starch, 2 Meat

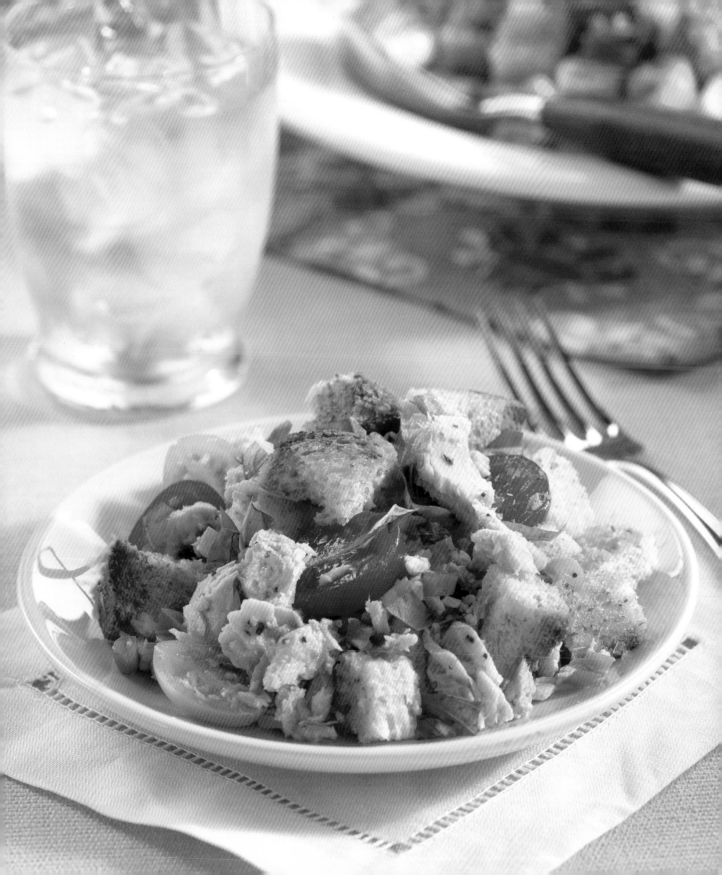

CHICKEN CAESAR SALAD WITH HOMEMADE CROUTONS

MAKES 4 SERVINGS

1. To make croutons, preheat oven to 350°F. Place bread cubes in gallon-size resealable bag. Drizzle with oil and 1/2 teaspoon seasoning. Seal bag; shake until bread is evenly coated with oil and seasoning. Spread bread cubes in single layer on baking sheet. Bake 12 to 15 minutes, turning 2 or 3 times during baking, until bread is just crisp (bread will continue to crisp as it cools). Remove from oven; set aside.

2. Prepare grill for direct cooking. Season chicken with remaining 1 teaspoon seasoning. Grill chicken over medium heat, covered, about 8 to 10 minutes, turning once, until chicken is no longer pink in center. Remove from grill. Let stand 5 minutes.

3. Meanwhile, in large bowl, toss together lettuce, dressing, cheese and croutons. Divide among four dinner plates. Cut chicken into strips and top each salad with chicken.

3 to 4 slices (3/4-inch-thick) whole grain artisan bread, cut into 3/4-inch cubes (about 2 cups)

2 tablespoons olive oil

1 1/2 teaspoons salt-free garlic-herb seasoning, divided

2 boneless skinless chicken breasts (4 ounces each)

8 cups torn romaine lettuce

1/4 cup fat-free Caesar dressing

1/3 cup shredded Parmesan cheese

Calories 270, **Total Fat** 12g, **Saturated Fat** 3g, **Cholesterol** 42mg, **Sodium** 564mg, **Carbohydrates** 22g, **Dietary Fiber** 3g, **Protein** 20g
Dietary Exchanges: 1 Bread/Starch, 2 Meat, 1 Vegetable, 1 Fat

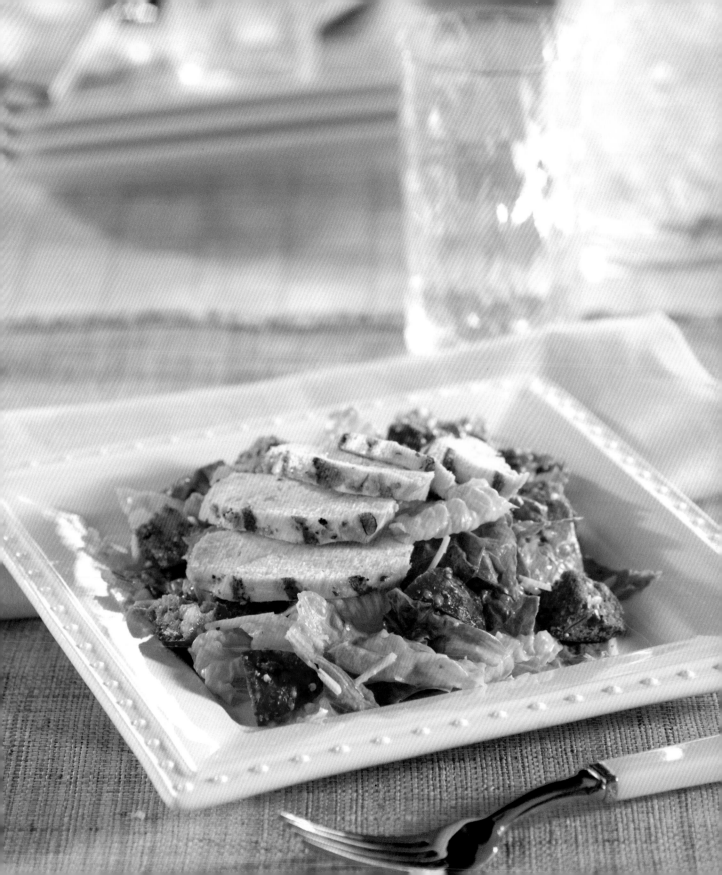

TURKEY AND SPINACH PANINIS WITH BASIL-DIJON AÏOLI

MAKES 4 SERVINGS

1. To make Aïoli, combine basil, mayonnaise, mustard and garlic in small bowl; set aside.

2. Meanwhile, remove soft portion of bread, leaving about $1/2$-inch-thick shell. Reserve bread pieces (about 4 ounces) for another use, such as for bread crumbs or croutons. (The "shell" should weigh 8 ounces.)

3. To assemble, sprinkle mozzarella cheese on bottom half of bread. Top with tomato, onion, turkey and spinach. Spread Aïoli on top portion of bread. Place on top; press down lightly to adhere.

4. Coat large skillet with nonstick cooking spray and place over medium heat. Place whole sandwich in skillet. Weigh down with a dinner plate. Cook 3 minutes on each side or until bread is golden and cheese is slightly melted. Cut into four pieces.

1 tablespoon dried basil

3 tablespoons light mayonnaise

1 tablespoon coarse-grain Dijon mustard

2 medium cloves garlic, minced

12 ounces whole-grain Italian loaf bread, cut in half lengthwise

3 ounces finely shredded part-skim mozzarella

1 medium tomato, thinly sliced

$1/2$ cup thinly sliced red onion

3 ounces thinly sliced oven-roasted turkey

1 to 2 ounces fresh baby spinach leaves

Calories 350, **Total Fat** 12g, **Saturated Fat** 3g, **Cholesterol** 28mg, **Sodium** 714mg, **Carbohydrates** 41g, **Dietary Fiber** 11g, **Protein** 21g
Dietary Exchanges: 3 Bread/Starch, 2 Meat, $1/2$ Fat

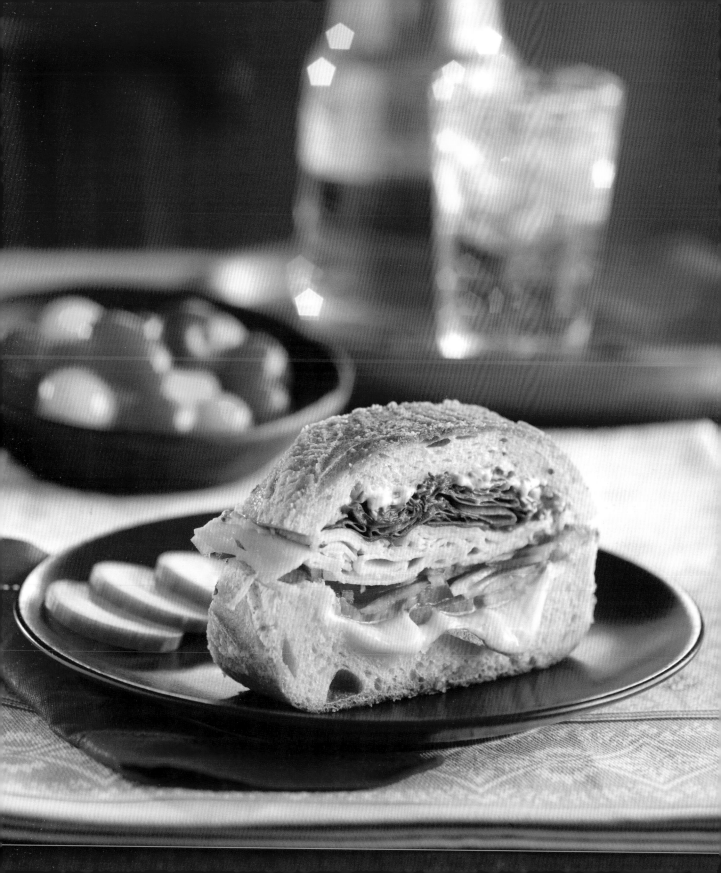

CHICKEN AND GINGER SPINACH SALAD

MAKES 4 SERVINGS

1. Combine dressing ingredients in small jar. Secure with lid; shake until well blended.

2. Bring water to a boil in large saucepan. Add peas; boil 30 seconds. Drain and immediately rinse under cold water to stop the cooking process.

3. To serve, arrange spinach on four plates. Top with onion, chicken, snow peas and strawberries. Sprinkle with nuts. Shake dressing; serve with salad.

DRESSING

1/3 cup fresh orange juice

1 tablespoon grated fresh ginger

3 tablespoons cider vinegar

3 tablespoons pourable sugar substitute*

1½ tablespoons canola oil

1/4 teaspoon red pepper flakes

1/4 teaspoon salt

SALAD

2 cups water

3 ounces fresh snow peas or sugar snap peas

6 ounces baby spinach (about 6 cups)

2 ounces sliced red onion (2-inch strips)

1 package (8½ ounces) diced cooked chicken breast (about 1¾ cups)

2 cups whole strawberries, quartered

1/4 cup (1 ounce) pistachio nuts or slivered almonds, toasted*

This recipe was tested using sucralose-based sugar substitute.

To toast pistachios, spread in single layer in heavy skillet. Cook over medium heat 1 to 2 minutes or until nuts are lightly browned, stirring frequently.

Calories 240, **Total Fat** 11g, **Saturated Fat** 1g, **Cholesterol** 46mg, **Sodium** 224mg, **Carbohydrates** 16g, **Dietary Fiber** 4g, **Protein** 22g
Dietary Exchanges: 2 Meat, 2 Vegetable, ½ Fruit, 1 Fat

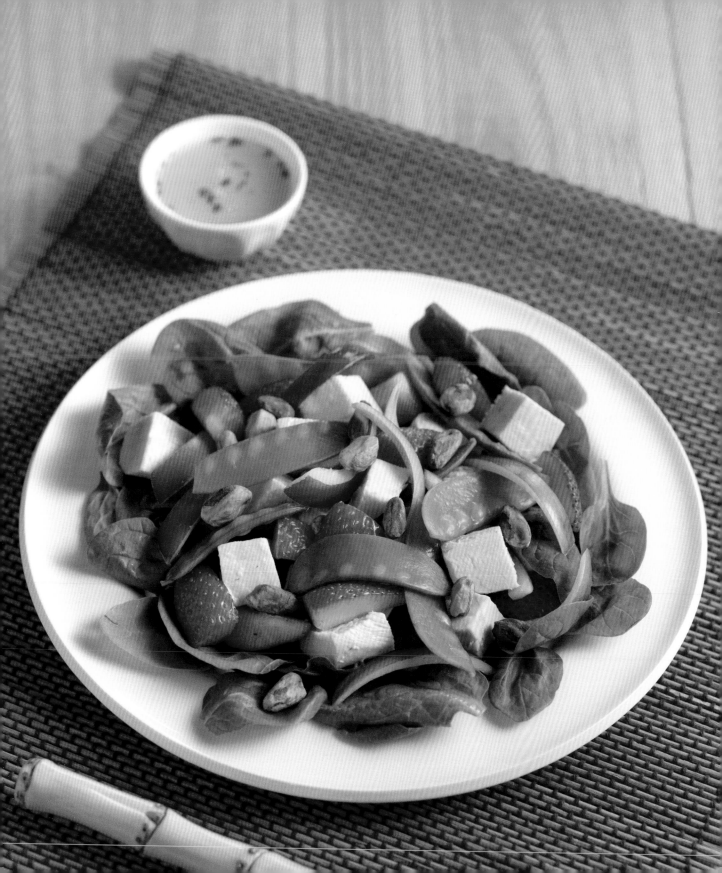

SOUTHWESTERN TUNA SALAD

MAKES 4 SERVINGS (1 CUP PER SERVING)

1. Place juice of one lime in glass baking dish or shallow bowl. Add tuna steaks. Marinate at room temperature 30 minutes, turning once.

2. Spray stovetop grill pan with nonstick cooking spray; heat over medium heat 30 seconds. Add tuna steaks; cook 5 to 6 minutes per side. Remove and set aside until cooled to room temperature. Cut into bite-size chunks.

3. Combine tomatoes, avocado, jalapeño pepper, green onion and cilantro in large bowl. Add tuna.

4. Whisk oil, remaining lime juice, salt, cumin and black pepper in small bowl. Pour over salad; toss to coat. Garnish with lime wedges, if desired.

2 limes, juiced, divided

12 ounces raw tuna steaks (about 1 inch thick)

1 pint cherry or grape tomatoes, halved

1/4 cup diced ripe avocado (1/4 of medium avocado)

1 jalapeño pepper,* seeded and minced

1 green onion, chopped (green parts only)

1 tablespoon chopped fresh cilantro

1 1/2 teaspoons canola oil

1/4 teaspoon salt

1/4 teaspoon ground cumin

1/8 teaspoon black pepper

Lime wedges (optional)

Jalapeño peppers can sting and irritate the skin, so wear rubber gloves when handling peppers and do not touch your eyes.

Calories 180, **Total Fat** 7g, **Saturated Fat** 2g, **Cholesterol** 30mg, **Sodium** 190mg, **Carbohydrates** 8g, **Dietary Fiber** 3g, **Protein** 21g
Dietary Exchanges: 3 Meat, 1 Vegetable

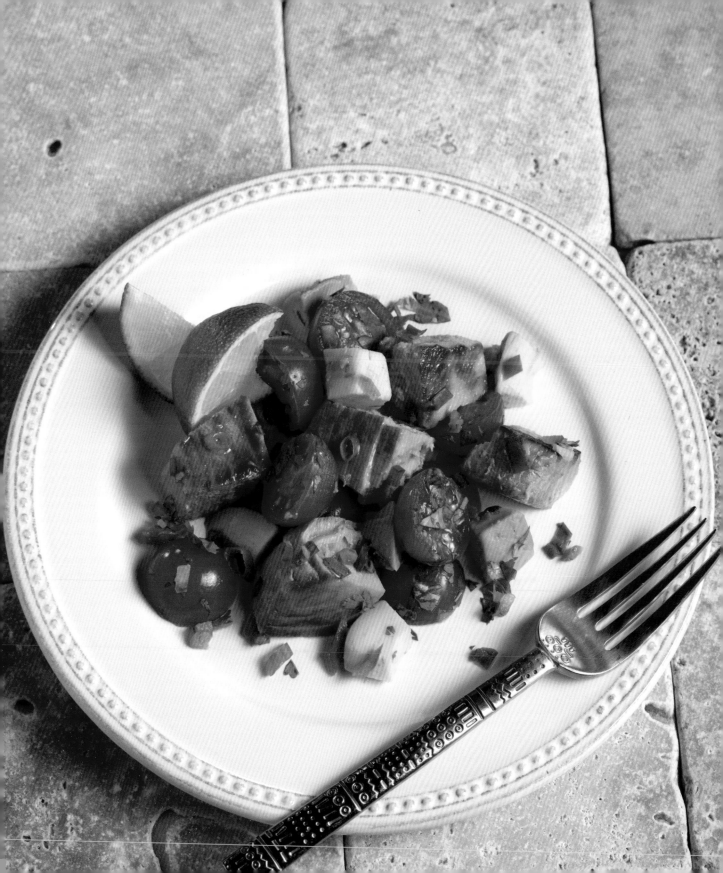

HEAVENLY CRANBERRY TURKEY SANDWICHES

MAKES 4 SERVINGS

1. Combine cream cheese and cranberry sauce in small bowl; mix well. Stir in walnuts.

2. Spread mixture on toast slices. Layer turkey and greens on four slices; top with remaining four slices. Cut diagonally in half.

1/4 cup reduced-fat cream cheese

1/4 cup cranberry sauce or chutney

2 tablespoons chopped toasted* walnuts

8 slices multigrain or whole wheat bread, lightly toasted

1/2 pound sliced deli smoked turkey breast

1 cup packed mesclun or spring salad mixed greens *or* 4 red leaf lettuce leaves

*To toast walnuts, spread in single layer on baking sheet. Bake in preheated 350°F oven 5 to 7 minutes or until fragrant, stirring occasionally.

Calories 291, **Total Fat** 8g, **Saturated Fat** 2g, **Cholesterol** 28mg, **Sodium** 698mg, **Carbohydrates** 39g, **Dietary Fiber** 9g, **Protein** 20g
Dietary Exchanges: 2 Bread/Starch, 2 Meat, 1/2 Fruit

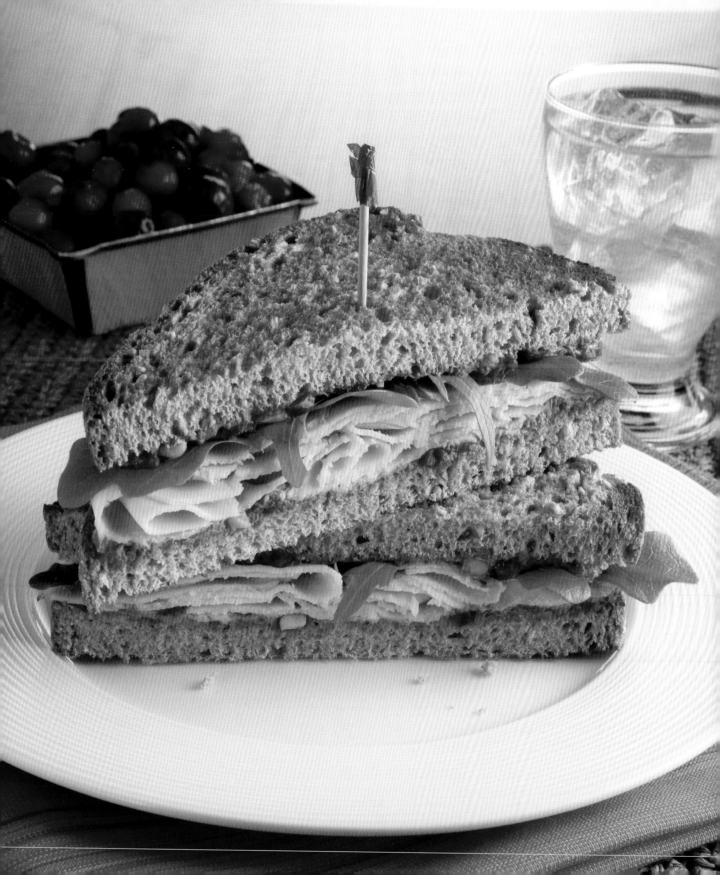

EGGPLANT AND FETA STUFFED PITAS

MAKES 6 SERVINGS

1. Heat oil in large nonstick skillet over medium-high heat. Add onion. Coat onion with nonstick cooking spray; cook 2 minutes. Add eggplant. Coat eggplant with cooking spray; cook 4 to 6 minutes or until beginning to lightly brown, stirring frequently. Add garlic; cook 15 seconds, stirring constantly. Add tomatoes; cook 2 minutes or until tomatoes are just tender.

2. Remove from heat; add basil. Cover; let stand 3 minutes to absorb flavors. To serve, spoon $1/3$ cup in each pita half; drizzle each with $1\frac{1}{2}$ teaspoons balsamic vinaigrette and sprinkle with $1\frac{1}{2}$ tablespoons feta.

- 2 teaspoons olive oil
- 1 cup diced onion
- $2\frac{1}{2}$ cups diced eggplant
- 1 clove garlic, minced
- 1 cup grape tomatoes, quartered
- $1/4$ cup chopped fresh basil
- 3 whole wheat pita bread rounds, warmed and halved
- $1/4$ cup reduced-fat balsamic vinaigrette
- 3 ounces crumbled reduced-fat feta cheese

Calories 162, **Total Fat** 5g, **Saturated Fat** 2g, **Cholesterol** 4mg, **Sodium** 526mg, **Carbohydrates** 25g, **Dietary Fiber** 5g, **Protein** 7g
Dietary Exchanges: 1 Bread/Starch, 1 Meat, 1 Vegetable, $1/2$ Fat

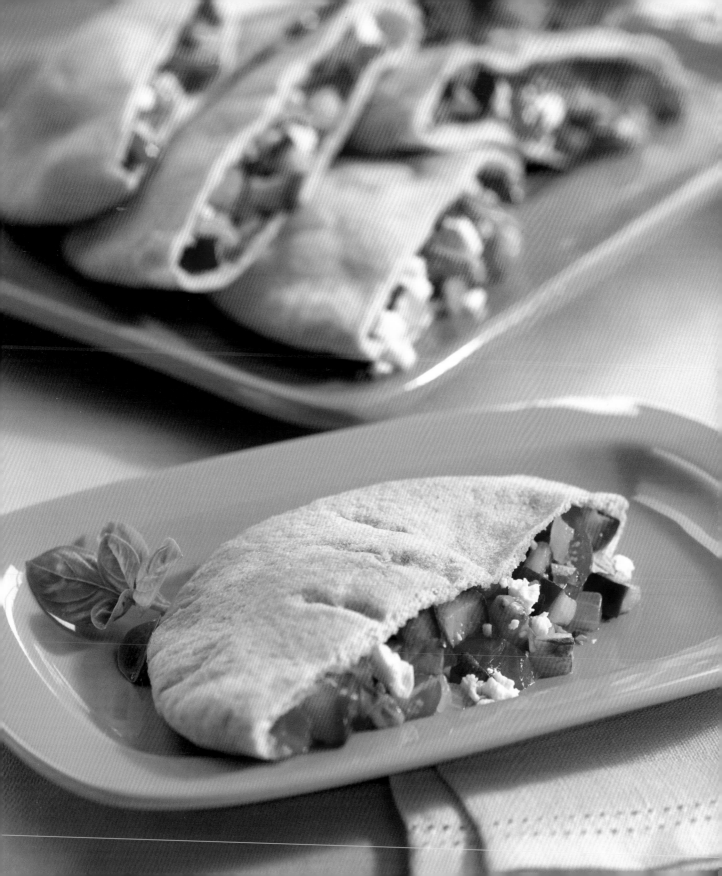

GREEK CHICKEN BURGERS WITH CUCUMBER YOGURT SAUCE

MAKES 4 SERVINGS (4-OUNCE BURGER AND 1/4 OF SAUCE PER SERVING)

1. Combine yogurt, cucumber, lemon juice, 2 cloves garlic, 2 teaspoons chopped mint, salt and white pepper in medium bowl; mix well. Cover and refrigerate until ready to serve.

2. Combine chicken, feta, olives, egg, oregano, black pepper and remaining 1 clove garlic in large bowl; mix well. Shape mixture into four patties.

3. Spray grill pan with nonstick cooking spray; heat over medium-high heat. Grill patties 5 to 7 minutes per side or until cooked through (165°F).

4. Serve burgers with sauce and mixed greens, if desired. Garnish with mint leaves.

1/2 cup plus 2 tablespoons plain nonfat Greek yogurt

1/2 medium cucumber, peeled, seeded and finely chopped

Juice of 1/2 lemon

3 cloves garlic, minced, divided

2 teaspoons finely chopped fresh mint *or* 1/2 teaspoon dried mint

1/8 teaspoon salt

1/8 teaspoon ground white pepper

1 pound ground chicken breast

3 ounces reduced-fat crumbled feta cheese

4 large kalamata olives, rinsed, patted dry and minced

1 egg, beaten

1/2 to 1 teaspoon dried oregano

1/4 teaspoon black pepper

Mixed baby lettuce (optional)

Fresh mint leaves (optional)

Calories 260, **Total Fat** 14g, **Saturated Fat** 5g, **Cholesterol** 150mg, **Sodium** 500mg, **Carbohydrates** 4g, **Dietary Fiber** 1g, **Protein** 29g
Dietary Exchanges: 3 Meat, 1/2 Vegetable, 1 Fat

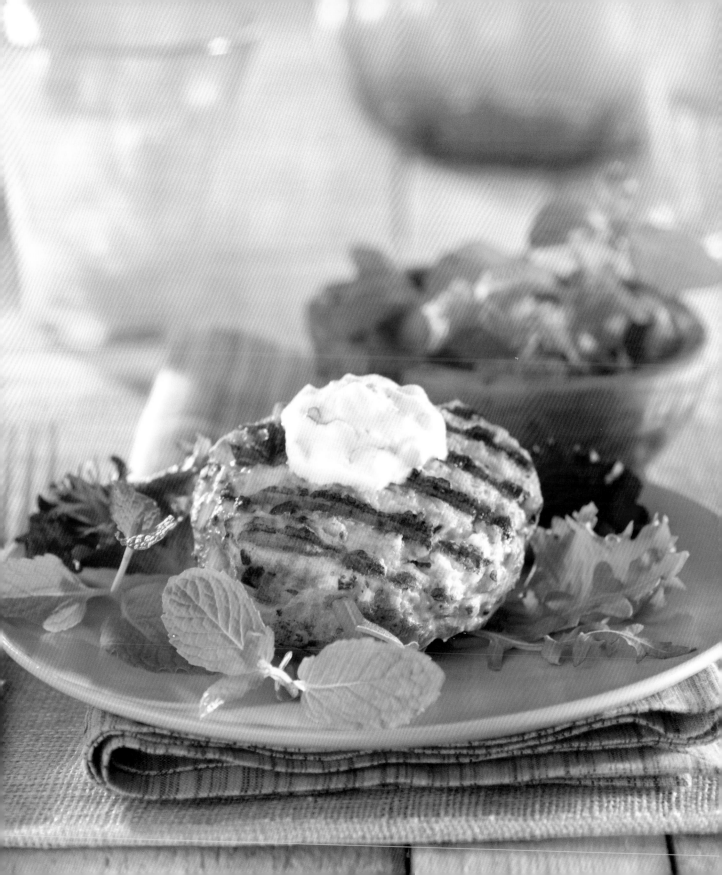

BBQ CHICKEN SALAD WITH ROASTED CORN AND CILANTRO

MAKES 4 SERVINGS (1 CUP PER SERVING)

1. Combine chicken, corn, red peppers, green onions and cilantro in large bowl; toss gently.

2. Combine oil, lime juice, mustard, black pepper and garlic in small bowl; whisk well.

3. Spoon dressing over chicken mixture; carefully toss to bind ingredients.

4. Divide salad mixture into four portions; spoon onto shredded cabbage, if desired.

2½ cups chopped cooked barbecue chicken*

½ cup corn, roasted**

3 to 4 canned sweet roasted red peppers, chopped

2 green onions, chopped

¼ cup fresh cilantro, minced

2 tablespoons canola oil

2 tablespoons lime juice

1 teaspoon Dijon mustard

⅛ teaspoon black pepper

1 clove garlic, minced

Shredded cabbage (optional)

*Purchase barbecue roasted chicken breasts from the deli and remove the skin.

**Roast whole ear of corn on grill or place under broiler until browned. Frozen or canned corn niblets can also be used.

Calories 196, **Total Fat** 12g, **Saturated Fat** 2g, **Cholesterol** 48mg, **Sodium** 289mg, **Carbohydrates** 11g, **Dietary Fiber** 1g, **Protein** 11g
Dietary Exchanges: 1 Bread/Starch, 1 Meat, 1½ Fat

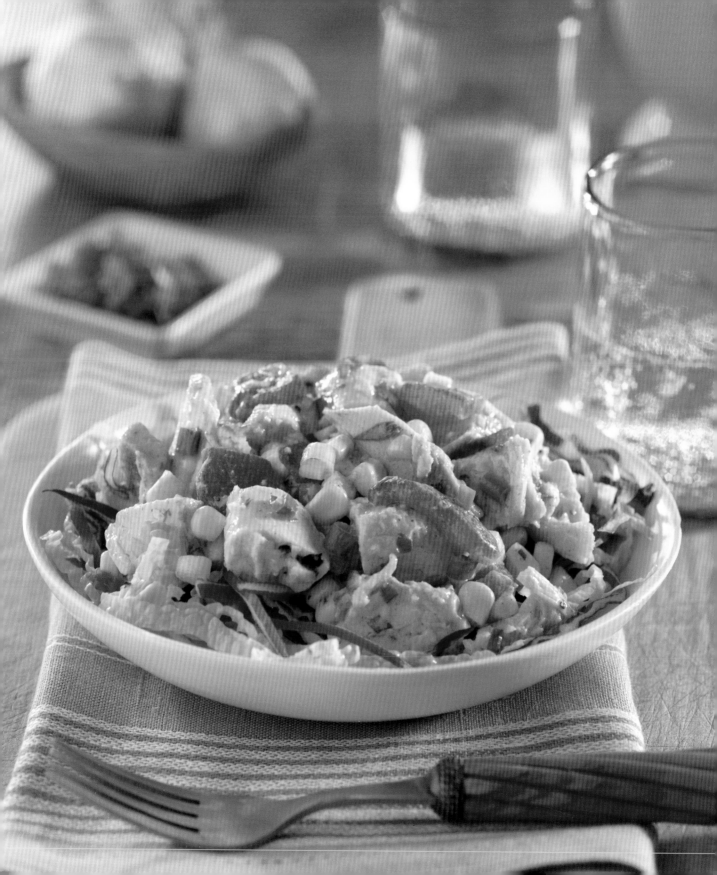

CHICKEN AND GRAPE PITA SANDWICHES

MAKES 6 SERVINGS

1. Bring 1 quart water to a boil in large saucepan. Add chicken; cover and remove from heat. Let stand 6 minutes or until chicken is cooked through (165°F). Drain. Rinse chicken under cold water; drain.

2. Stir yogurt, mayonnaise, tarragon, mustard, honey and pepper in large bowl until well blended. Add chicken, celery and grapes; toss to coat evenly. Separate lettuce leaves. Select six large leaves and discard stems. Tear or shred remaining leaves.

3. Line each pita half with whole lettuce leaf. Fill with handful of torn lettuce leaves and about $2/3$ cup chicken mixture.

1 pound boneless skinless chicken breasts, cut into $1/2$-inch pieces

$1/2$ cup plain nonfat yogurt

$1/4$ cup reduced-fat mayonnaise

2 tablespoons fresh tarragon leaves, minced, *or* 2 teaspoons dried tarragon leaves

2 teaspoons Dijon mustard

2 teaspoons honey

$1/2$ teaspoon black pepper

1 cup thinly sliced celery

1 cup red seedless grapes, cut into halves

1 medium head red leaf lettuce, washed

3 pita bread rounds, cut in half crosswise

Calories 249, **Total Fat** 6g, **Saturated Fat** 1g, **Cholesterol** 50mg, **Sodium** 278mg, **Carbohydrates** 28g, **Dietary Fiber** 1g, **Protein** 22g
Dietary Exchanges: 1 Bread/Starch, 2 Meat, $2^{1}/_{2}$ Vegetable

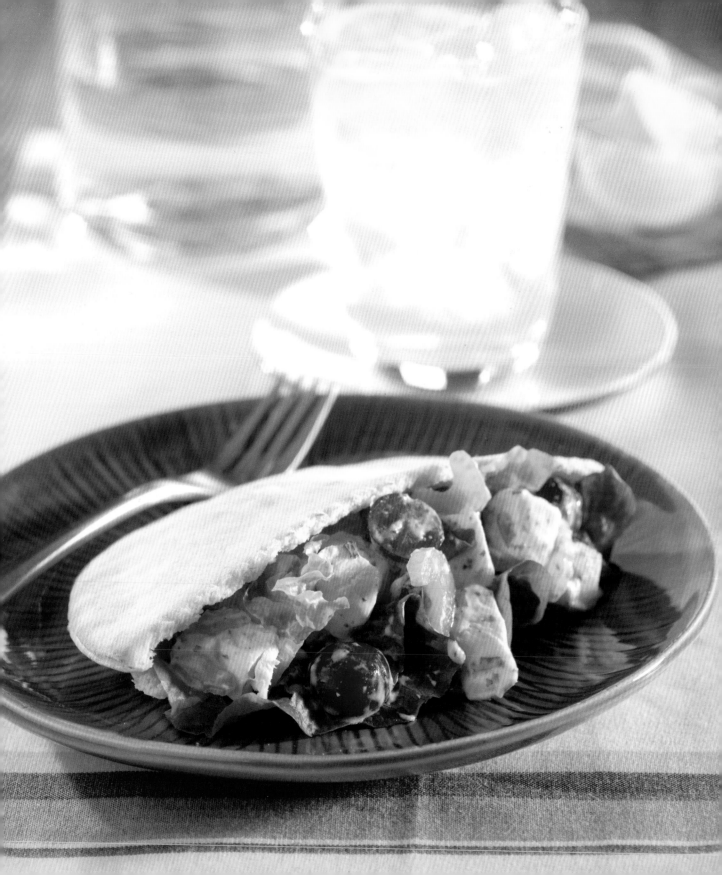

SCALLOP AND SPINACH SALAD

MAKES 4 SERVINGS

1. Pat spinach dry; place in large bowl with red onion. Cover; set aside.

2. Rinse scallops. Cut in half horizontally (to make 2 thin rounds); pat dry. Sprinkle top sides lightly with red pepper and paprika. Spray large nonstick skillet with nonstick cooking spray; heat over high heat until very hot. Add half of scallops, seasoned sides down, in single layer, placing $1/2$ inch or more apart. Cook 2 minutes or until browned on bottom. Turn scallops; cook 1 to 2 minutes or until opaque in center. Transfer to plate; cover to keep warm. Wipe skillet clean; repeat procedure with remaining scallops.

3. Place dressing in small saucepan; bring to a boil over high heat. Pour dressing over spinach and onion; toss to coat. Divide among four plates. Place scallops on top of spinach; sprinkle with blue cheese and walnuts.

1 package (10 ounces) fresh spinach leaves, washed, stemmed and torn

3 thin slices red onion, halved and separated

12 ounces sea scallops

$1/8$ teaspoon ground red pepper

$1/8$ teaspoon paprika

$1/2$ cup fat-free Italian salad dressing

$1/4$ cup crumbled blue cheese

2 tablespoons toasted walnuts

Calories 169, **Total Fat** 6g, **Saturated Fat** 2g, **Cholesterol** 50mg, **Sodium** 660mg, **Carbohydrates** 6g, **Dietary Fiber** 2g, **Protein** 24g
Dietary Exchanges: 3 Meat, 1 Vegetable

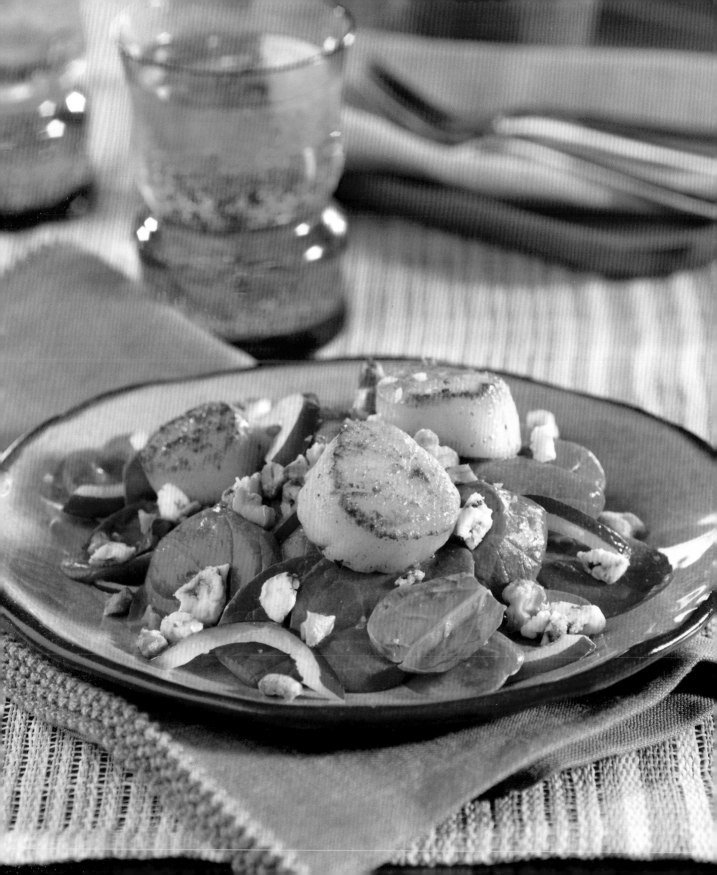

SWEET AND SOUR BROCCOLI PASTA SALAD

MAKES 6 SERVINGS

1. Cook pasta according to package directions, omitting salt. Add broccoli during the last 2 minutes of cooking; drain. Rinse under cold running water until pasta and broccoli are cool.

2. Combine pasta, broccoli, carrots and apple in medium bowl.

3. Whisk yogurt, apple juice, vinegar, oil, mustard, honey and thyme in small bowl until smooth and well blended. Pour over pasta mixture; toss to coat.

4. Line six plates with lettuce. Top evenly with pasta salad.

8 ounces uncooked pasta twists

2 cups broccoli florets

$2/3$ cup shredded carrots

1 medium Red or Golden Delicious apple, cored, seeded and chopped

$1/3$ cup plain nonfat yogurt

$1/3$ cup apple juice

3 tablespoons cider vinegar

1 tablespoon olive oil

1 tablespoon Dijon mustard

1 teaspoon honey

$1/2$ teaspoon dried thyme

Lettuce leaves

Calories 198, **Total Fat** 3g, **Saturated Fat** 1g, **Cholesterol** 1mg, **Sodium** 57mg, **Carbohydrates** 36g, **Dietary Fiber** 3g, **Protein** 7g
Dietary Exchanges: 2 Bread/Starch, $1/2$ Vegetable, $1/2$ Fruit, $1/2$ Fat

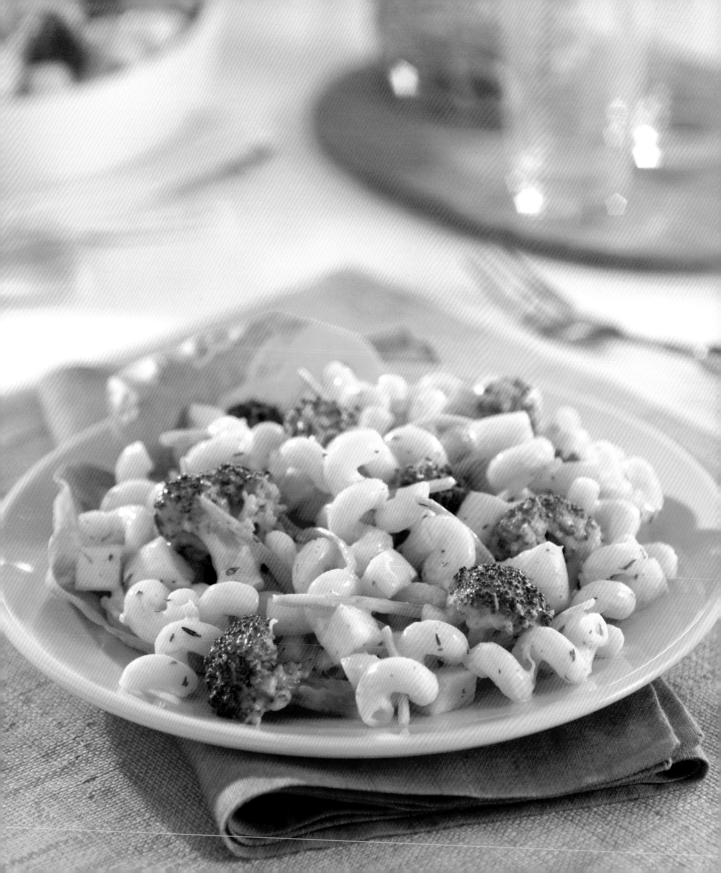

RASPBERRY MANGO SALAD

MAKES 4 SERVINGS

1. Combine arugula, lettuce, mango, raspberries, watercress and cheese in medium bowl.

2. Place water, oil, vinegar, salt and pepper in small jar; shake to combine. Pour over salad; toss to coat. Serve immediately.

2 cups baby spinach or arugula

1 cup torn Bibb or Boston lettuce

1 cup diced peeled mango (about 1)

$3/4$ cup fresh raspberries

$1/2$ cup stemmed watercress

$1/4$ cup ($1^1/2$ ounces) crumbled blue cheese

1 tablespoon water

1 tablespoon olive oil

1 tablespoon raspberry vinegar

$1/8$ teaspoon salt

$1/8$ teaspoon black pepper

Calories 98, **Total Fat** 8g, **Saturated Fat** 3g, **Cholesterol** 8mg, **Sodium** 227mg, **Carbohydrates** 12g, **Dietary Fiber** 2g, **Protein** 3g
Dietary Exchanges: 2 Vegetable, 2 Fat

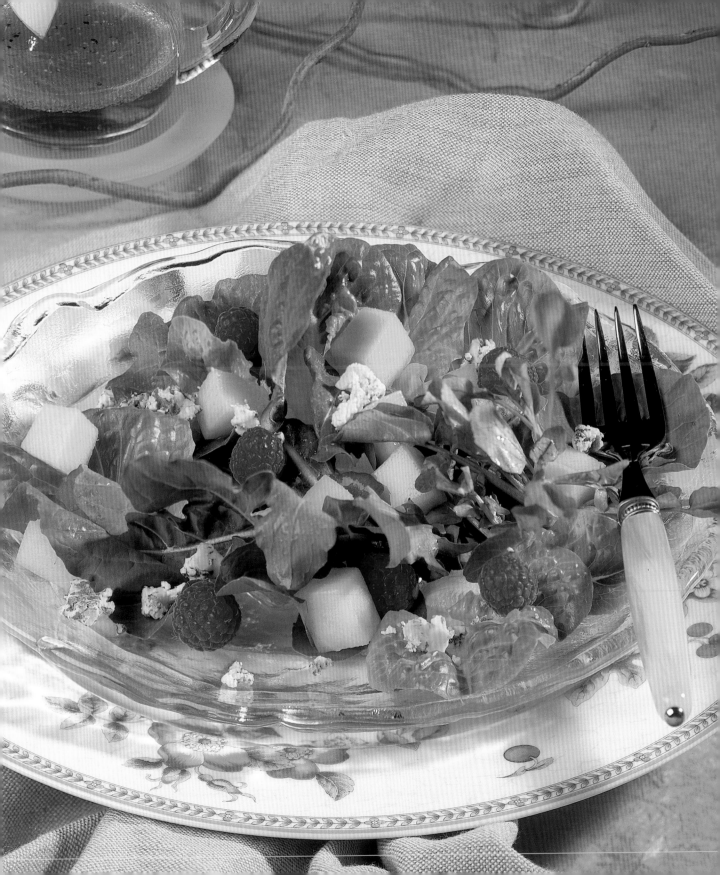

FARRO, CHICKPEA & SPINACH SALAD

MAKES 6 SERVINGS

1. Bring 4 cups water to a boil in medium saucepan. Add farro; reduce heat and simmer 20 to 25 minutes or until farro is tender. Drain and rinse under cold water until cool.

2. Meanwhile, combine spinach, cucumber, chickpeas, olives, oil, vinegar, rosemary, garlic, salt and red pepper flakes, if desired, in large bowl. Stir in farro until well blended. Add cheese; stir gently.

$3/4$ cup uncooked pearled farro

3 cups baby spinach, stemmed

1 medium cucumber, chopped

1 can (about 15 ounces) chickpeas, rinsed and drained

$1/2$ cup pitted kalamata olives

$1/4$ cup extra virgin olive oil

3 tablespoons white or golden balsamic vingar or 3 tablespoons cider vinegar mixed with $1/2$ teaspoon sugar

1 teaspoon chopped fresh rosemary

1 clove garlic, minced

$1/8$ to $1/4$ teaspoon red pepper flakes (optional)

$1/4$ cup crumbled goat or feta cheese

Calories 190, **Total Fat** 9g, **Saturated Fat** 1.5g, **Cholesterol** 5mg, **Sodium** 210mg, **Carbohydrates** 22g, **Dietary Fiber** 4g, **Protein** 6g
Dietary Exchanges: 1 Bread/Starch, $1/2$ Vegetable, $1^1/2$ Fat

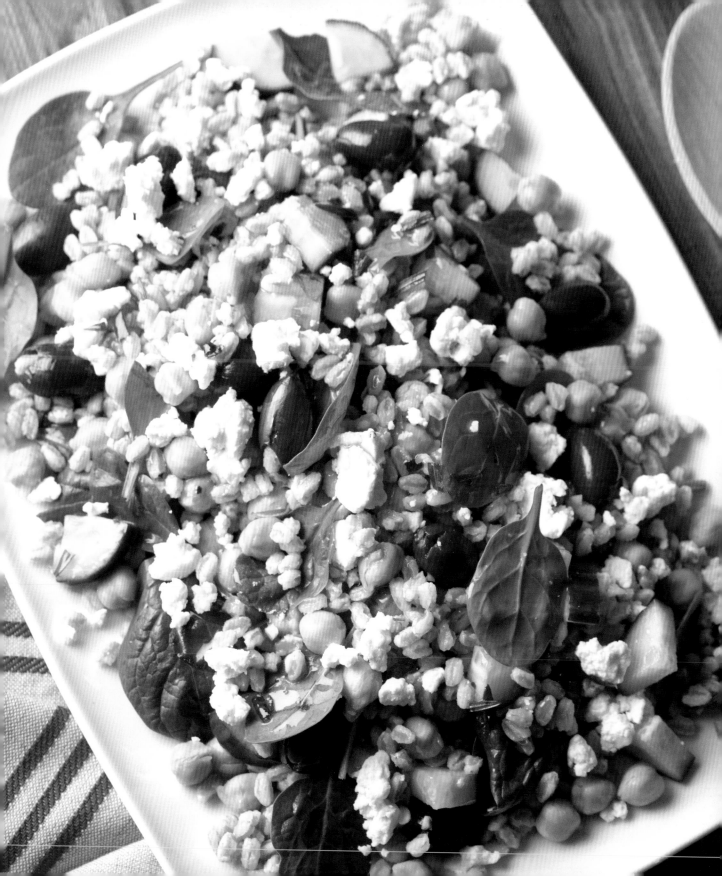

GRILLED PORTOBELLO MUSHROOM SANDWICH

MAKES 1 SERVING

1. Brush mushroom, bell pepper, onion and cut sides of bun lightly with dressing; set bun aside. Place vegetables over medium-hot coals. Grill 2 minutes.

2. Turn vegetables; brush with dressing. Grill 2 minutes or until vegetables are tender. Remove bell pepper and onion from grill.

3. Place bun halves, cut sides down, on grill. Turn mushroom top side up; brush with any remaining dressing; top with cheese. Grill 1 minute or until cheese is melted and bun is lightly toasted.

4. Cut pepper into strips. Place mushroom on bottom half of bun; top with onion slice and pepper strips. Cover with top half of bun.

NOTE: To broil, brush mushroom, bell pepper, onion and cut sides of bun with dressing. Place vegetables on greased rack of broiler pan; set bun aside. Broil vegetables 4 to 6 inches from heat 3 minutes; turn. Brush with dressing. Broil 3 minutes or until vegetables are tender. Place mushroom, top side up, on broiler pan; top with cheese. Place bun, cut sides up, on broiler pan. Broil 1 minute or until cheese is melted and bun is toasted. Assemble sandwich as directed above.

1 large portobello mushroom, cleaned and stemmed

1/4 medium green bell pepper, halved

1 thin slice red onion

1 whole wheat hamburger bun, split

2 tablespoons fat-free Italian salad dressing

1 slice (1 ounce) reduced-fat part-skim mozzarella cheese

Calories 225, **Total Fat** 6g, **Saturated Fat** 3g, **Cholesterol** 27mg, **Sodium** 729mg, **Carbohydrates** 30g, **Dietary Fiber** 6g, **Protein** 15g
Dietary Exchanges: 2 Bread/Starch, 1 Meat, 1/2 Fat

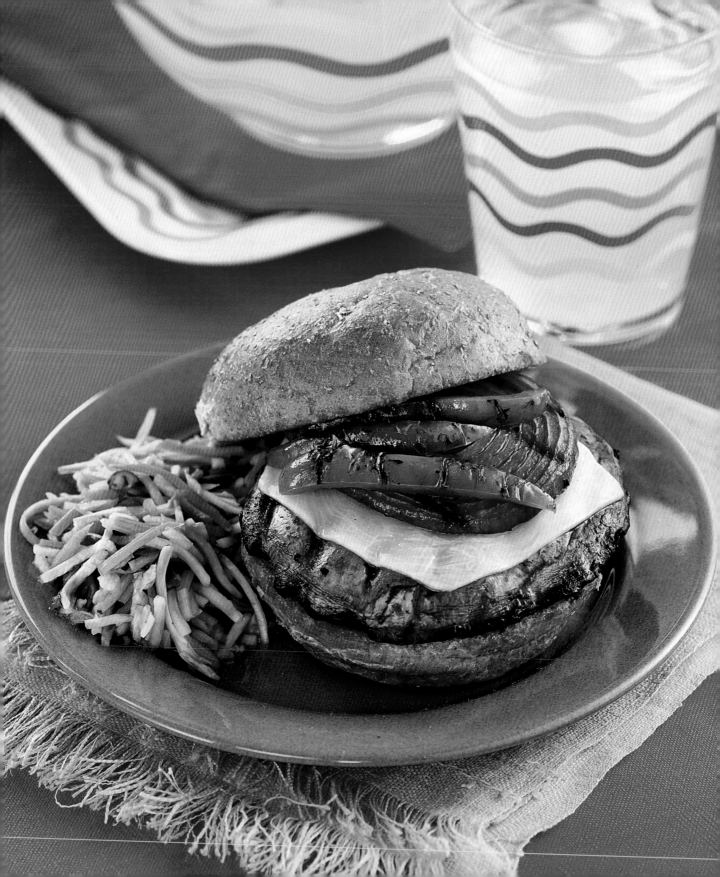

TUNA MELTS

MAKES 4 SERVINGS

1. Preheat broiler. Combine tuna, coleslaw mix and green onions in medium bowl. Combine mayonnaise, mustard and dill weed, if desired, in small bowl. Stir mayonnaise mixture into tuna mixture. Spread tuna mixture onto muffin halves. Place on broiler pan.

2. Broil 4 inches from heat 3 to 4 minutes or until heated through. Sprinkle with cheese. Broil 1 to 2 minutes more or until cheese is melted.

1 can (12 ounces) reduced-sodium chunk white tuna packed in water, drained and flaked

1½ cups packaged coleslaw mix

3 tablespoons sliced green onions

3 tablespoons reduced-fat mayonnaise

1 tablespoon Dijon mustard

1 teaspoon dried dill weed (optional)

4 English muffins, split and lightly toasted

⅓ cup shredded reduced-fat Cheddar cheese

Calories 294, **Total Fat** 6g, **Saturated Fat** 1g, **Cholesterol** 31mg, **Sodium** 459mg, **Carbohydrates** 29g, **Dietary Fiber** 2g, **Protein** 29g
Dietary Exchanges: 2 Bread/Starch, 3 Meat

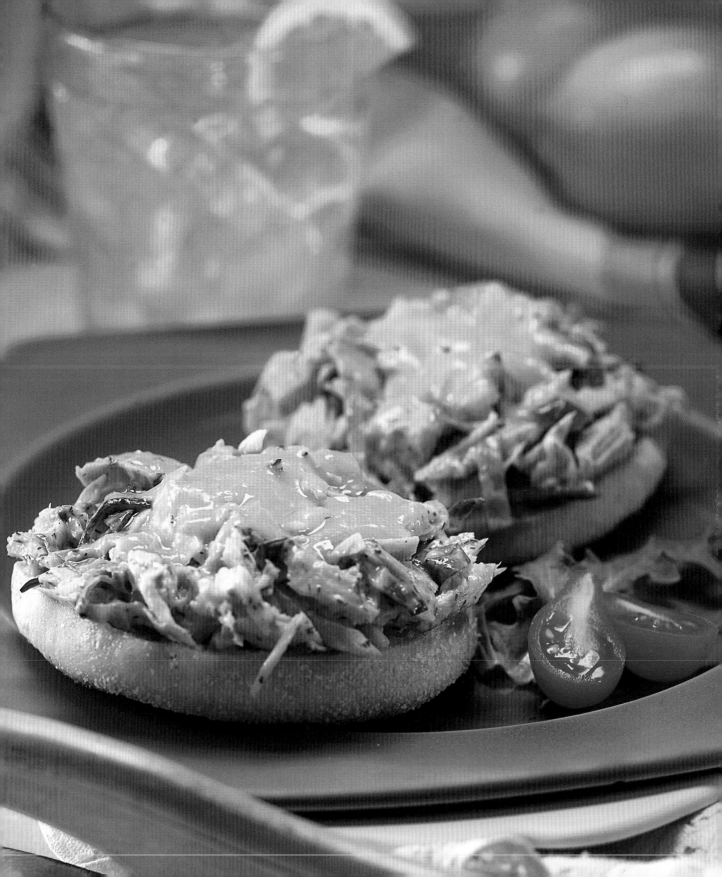

TOASTED PEANUT COUSCOUS SALAD

MAKES 4 SERVINGS

1. Bring water to a boil in small saucepan over high heat. Remove from heat; stir in couscous. Cover tightly and let stand 5 minutes or until water is absorbed. Place in medium bowl; cool slightly. Stir in onion and bell pepper.

2. Heat small nonstick skillet over medium-high heat until hot. Add peanuts; cook 2 to 3 minutes or until beginning to turn golden, stirring frequently. Add to couscous.

3. Whisk soy sauce, vinegar, oil, ginger, sugar substitute, salt and red pepper flakes in small bowl. Add to couscous; stir until well blended.

$1/2$ **cup water**

$1/4$ **cup uncooked couscous**

$1/2$ **cup finely chopped red onion**

$1/2$ **cup finely chopped green bell pepper**

1 **ounce unsalted dry-roasted peanuts**

1 **tablespoon reduced-sodium soy sauce**

2 **teaspoons cider vinegar**

$1^{1/2}$ **teaspoons sesame oil**

$1/2$ **teaspoon grated fresh ginger**

1 **packet sugar substitute***

$1/4$ **teaspoon salt**

$1/8$ **teaspoon red pepper flakes**

This recipe was tested using sucralose-based sugar substitute.

Calories 115, **Total Fat** 5g, **Saturated Fat** 1g, **Cholesterol** 0mg, **Sodium** 298mg, **Carbohydrates** 14g, **Dietary Fiber** 2g, **Protein** 4g
Dietary Exchanges: 1 Bread/Starch, 1 Fat

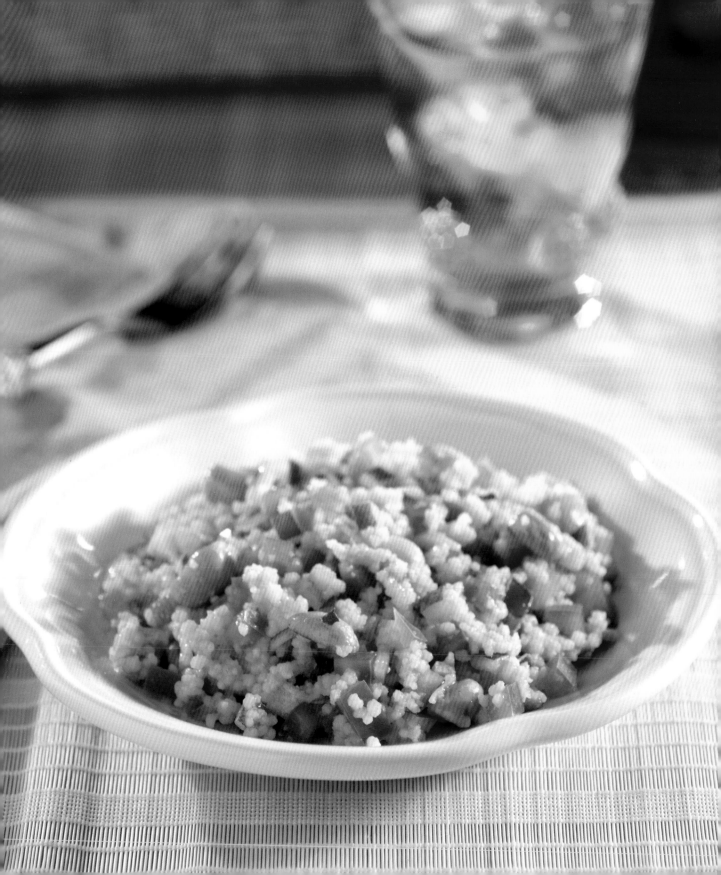

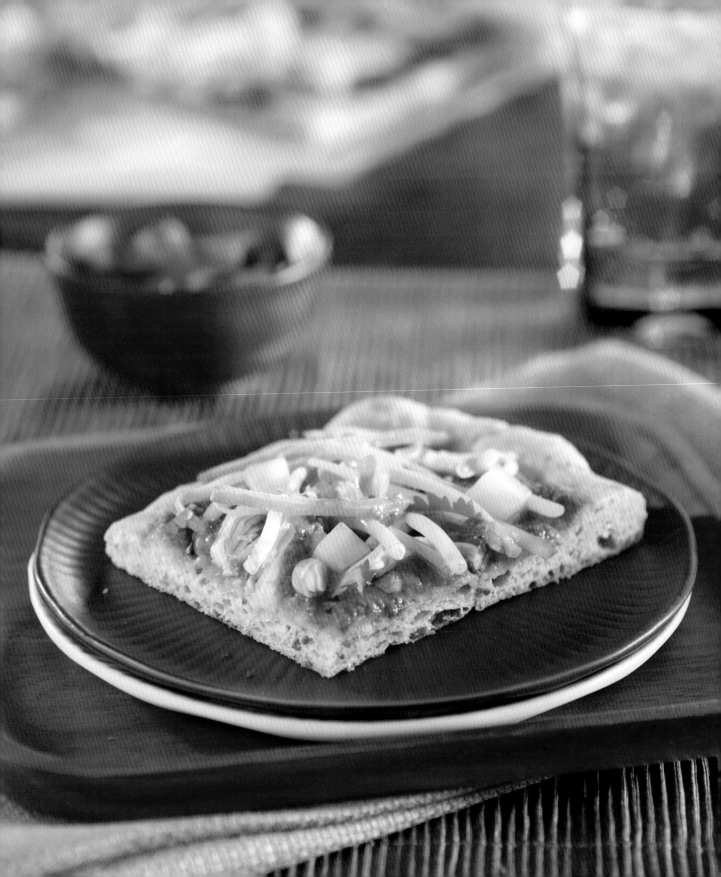

NOURISHING DINNERS

THAI CHICKEN PIZZA

MAKES 6 SERVINGS

1. Preheat oven to 450°F. Place pizza crust on baking sheet. Spread peanut sauce in thin layer over crust within 1/2-inch of edge. Sprinkle with cilantro. Arrange chicken evenly over crust. Bake 8 minutes or until warm.

2. Sprinkle cucumber, bean sprouts, carrots and green onion over top of pizza. Cut into wedges and top with cilantro, if desired.

1 package (10 ounces) ready-made whole wheat pizza crust

1/4 cup peanut sauce

1/3 cup chopped fresh cilantro

1 1/4 cups (4 ounces) shredded cooked chicken

1/2 cup diced cucumber

3/4 cup fresh or canned bean sprouts, rinsed and drained

3/4 cup shredded or matchstick carrots

1/3 cup sliced green onion

Chopped fresh cilantro (optional)

Calories 220, **Total Fat** 5g, **Saturated Fat** 2g, **Cholesterol** 22mg, **Sodium** 418mg, **Carbohydrates** 30g, **Dietary Fiber** 6g, **Protein** 15g
Dietary Exchanges: 2 Bread/Starch, 1 Meat

VEGETARIAN PAELLA

MAKES 6 SERVINGS

1. Heat oil in large nonstick skillet over medium-high heat. Add onion and garlic; cook 6 to 7 minutes or until onion is translucent. Reduce heat to medium-low. Stir in rice; cook and stir 1 minute.

2. Add broth, Italian seasoning, salt, if desired, turmeric and ground red pepper. Bring to a boil. Cover and simmer 30 minutes.

3. Stir in tomatoes, bell pepper and carrots. Cover and simmer 10 minutes.

4. Reduce heat to low. Stir in artichoke hearts, zucchini and peas. Cover and cook 10 minutes or until vegetables are crisp-tender.

2 teaspoons canola oil

1 cup chopped onion

2 cloves garlic, minced

1 cup uncooked brown rice

2¼ cups vegetable broth

1 teaspoon Italian seasoning

¾ teaspoon salt (optional)

½ teaspoon ground turmeric

⅛ teaspoon ground red pepper

1 can (about 14 ounces) no-salt-added stewed tomatoes

1 cup chopped red bell pepper

1 cup coarsely chopped carrots

1 can (14 ounces) quartered artichoke hearts, drained

1 small zucchini, halved lengthwise and sliced to ¼-inch thickness (about 1¼ cups)

½ cup frozen baby peas

Calories 241, **Total Fat** 7g, **Saturated Fat** 1g, **Cholesterol** 0mg, **Sodium** 470mg, **Carbohydrates** 43g, **Dietary Fiber** 7g, **Protein** 5g
Dietary Exchanges: 3 Bread/Starch, 1 Fat

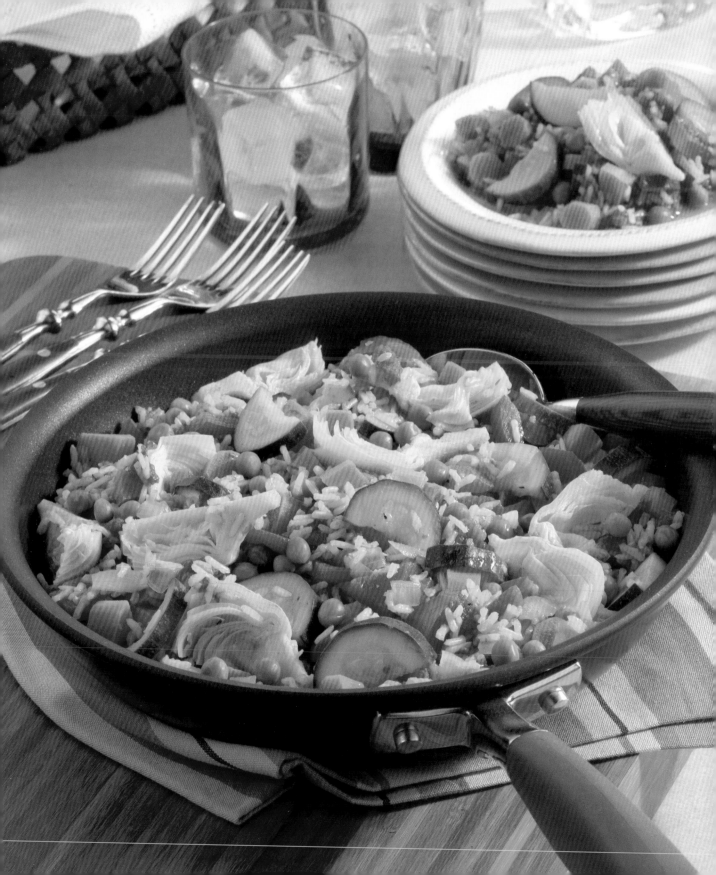

CHIPOTLE SHRIMP WITH SQUASH RIBBONS

MAKES 4 SERVINGS (1¼ CUPS PER SERVING)

1. Place garlic cloves, chipotle pepper in adobo sauce and water in food processor; purée until smooth.

2. Using a vegetable peeler, shave squash into ribbons (discarding the seedy middle). Set aside.

3. Heat oil in large skillet over high heat; add onion and bell pepper. Cook and stir 1 minute. Add shrimp and chipotle mixture; cook an additional 2 minutes. Add squash; cook and stir constantly 1 to 2 minutes or until shrimp are no longer pink and squash are heated through and slightly wilted. Garnish with lime wedges, if desired.

NOTE: Chipotle peppers are smoked jalapeños. They're usually found canned with adobo sauce, which is a dark red Mexican-style sauce made of chili peppers, herbs and vinegar. You can freeze leftovers in a food-safe container for later use.

2 cloves garlic

1 canned chipotle pepper in adobo sauce, plus 1 teaspoon sauce

2 tablespoons water

2 medium zucchini

2 medium yellow squash

1 teaspoon olive oil

1 small onion, diced

1 medium red bell pepper, cut into strips

½ pound raw medium shrimp, peeled and deveined

Lime wedges (optional)

Calories 139, **Total Fat** 3g, **Saturated Fat** 1g, **Cholesterol** 86mg, **Sodium** 111mg, **Carbohydrates** 13g, **Dietary Fiber** 3g, **Protein** 14g
Dietary Exchanges: 2 Meat, 2 Vegetable

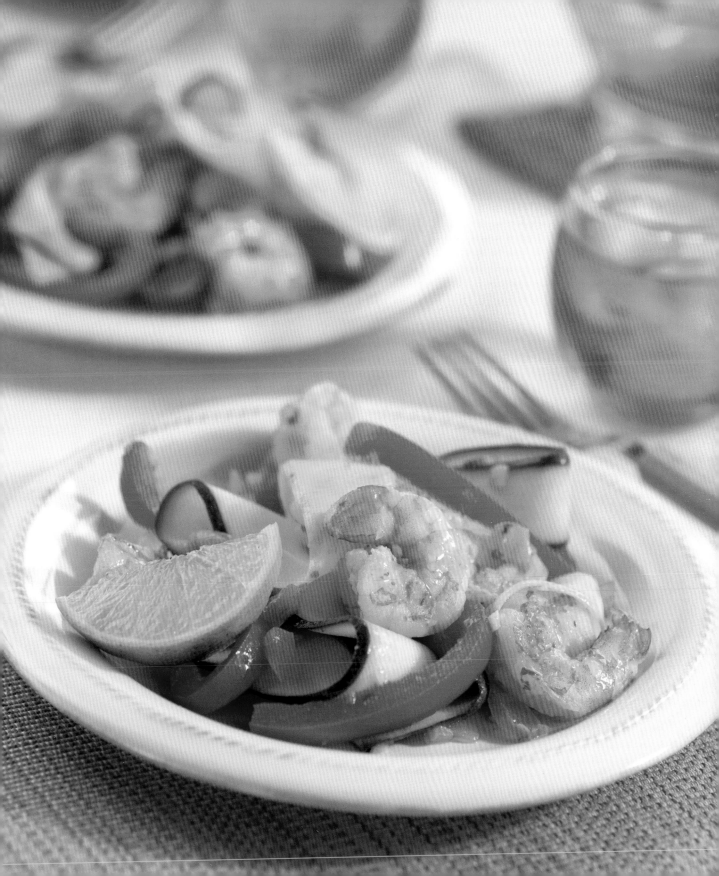

COUSCOUS-SPINACH-STUFFED PEPPERS

MAKES 4 SERVINGS (1 STUFFED PEPPER AND $1/4$ CUP SAUCE PER SERVING)

1. Heat large nonstick skillet over medium-high heat. Add couscous; lightly roast about 5 minutes, stirring occasionally. Remove onto plate; set aside.

2. In same skillet, heat oil. Add onion; cook 2 to 3 minutes until onion is translucent. Add spinach, oregano and salt; cook and stir 1 to 2 minutes until spinach is wilted. Add 2 cups water, bring to a boil. Stir in couscous; return to a boil. Reduce heat to a simmer; cover and cook 7 to 8 minutes until water is absorbed.

3. Cut off $1/2$ inch from tops of bell peppers; remove seeds and membranes. Fill peppers with couscous mixture; cover with tops. Place peppers in deep skillet that holds peppers upright. Add $1/4$ cup water to bottom of skillet. Bring water to a boil over medium-high heat; cover tightly with lid. Cook 8 to 9 minutes until peppers are slightly soft. Remove peppers to serving dish.

4. Meanwhile, place sauce ingredients in food processor. Cover; process until smooth. Transfer to small microwave-safe plate. Microwave on HIGH 2 minutes, stirring once. Serve sauce with peppers.

$3/4$ cup uncooked regular or whole wheat French couscous

1 tablespoon canola oil

$1/2$ cup finely chopped onion

3 cups (4 ounces) fresh spinach, chopped *or* 4 ounces frozen spinach, chopped

1 teaspoon dried oregano

$1/2$ teaspoon salt

$2^1/4$ cups water, divided

4 medium bell peppers, any color

SAUCE

$1/2$ cup roasted bell peppers

$1/2$ cup tomato sauce

$1/2$ teaspoon ground red pepper (optional)

Calories 213, **Total Fat** 4g, **Saturated Fat** 1g, **Cholesterol** 0mg, **Sodium** 522mg, **Carbohydrates** 38g, **Dietary Fiber** 5g, **Protein** 7g
Dietary Exchanges: $2^1/2$ Bread/Starch, $1/2$ Fat

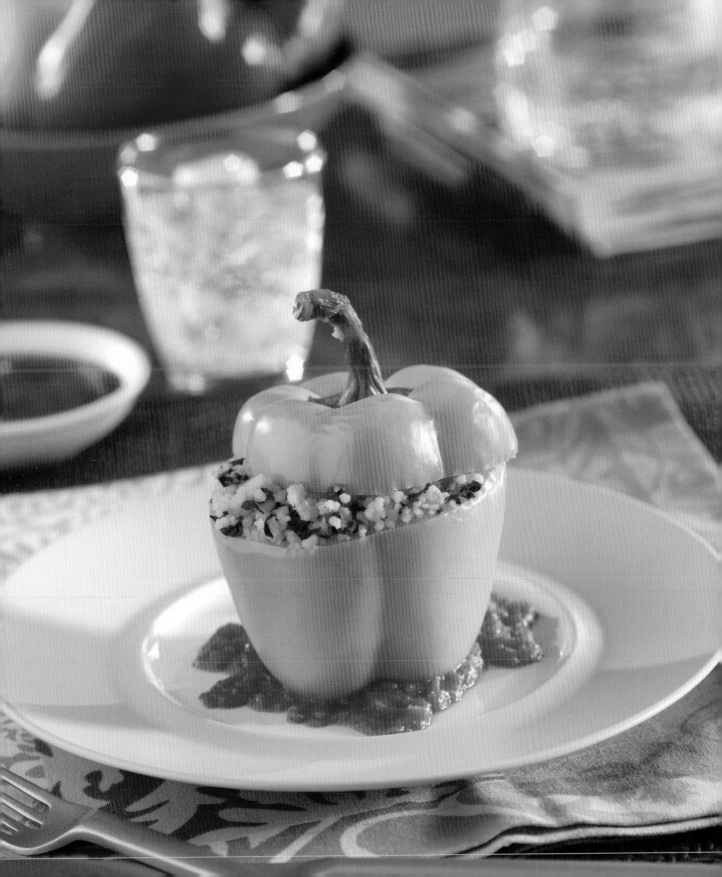

SIRLOIN STEAK WITH VEGETABLE SALAD

MAKES 4 SERVINGS (3 OUNCES COOKED BEEF
AND ABOUT ¾ CUP VEGETABLE SALAD PER SERVING)

1. Spray large skillet with nonstick cooking spray; heat over medium-high heat. Add bell pepper; cook 2 to 3 minutes. Add squash and onion; cook 5 minutes on each side or until just crisp-tender. Remove vegetables and place on large cutting board.

2. Sprinkle both sides of beef with steak seasoning and salt. Add beef to skillet; cook 4 minutes on each side or to desired degree of doneness. Remove to cutting board; let stand 3 minutes before thinly slicing.

3. Meanwhile, coarsely chop vegetables and place in medium bowl.

4. Toss vegetables with tomatoes and salad dressing. Add cheese and toss gently. Serve alongside beef slices.

- 1 medium red bell pepper, quartered
- 1 medium yellow squash, halved lengthwise
- 1 medium onion, halved and separated
- 1 boneless beef top sirloin steak (about 1 pound)
- 1½ teaspoons salt-free steak seasoning
- ¼ teaspoon salt
- ½ cup grape tomatoes, halved
- ¼ cup reduced-fat vinaigrette salad dressing
- ¼ cup crumbled blue cheese

Calories 248, **Total Fat** 10g, **Saturated Fat** 3g, **Cholesterol** 53mg, **Sodium** 426mg, **Carbohydrates** 9g, **Dietary Fiber** 2g, **Protein** 28g
Dietary Exchanges: 3 Meat, 2 Vegetable, 1 Fat

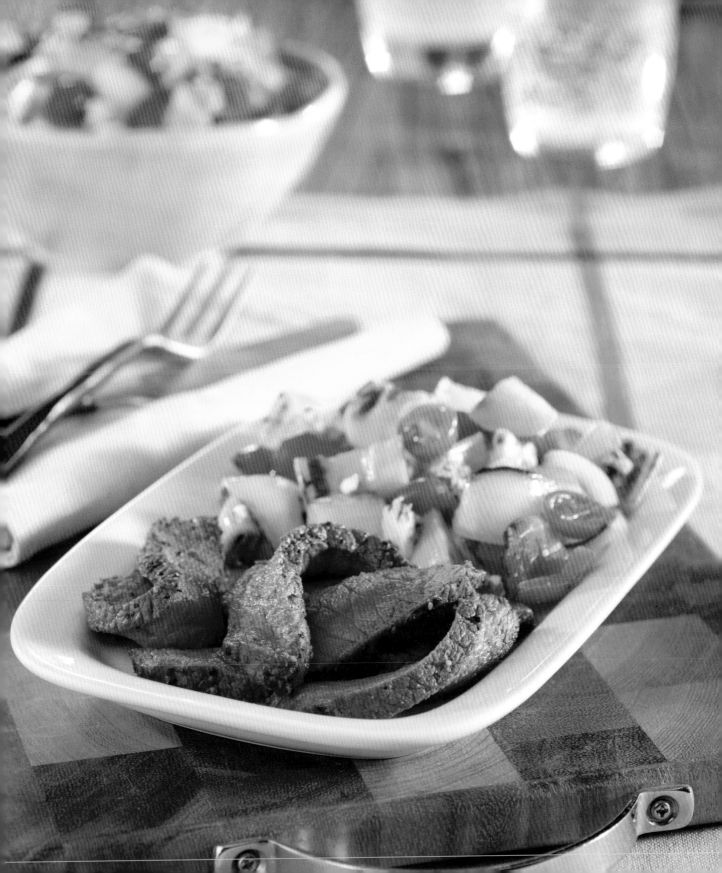

GARLIC GRILLED BEEF BROCHETTES

MAKES 4 SERVINGS

1. Preheat grill to medium-high heat. Combine dressing and garlic in shallow dish. Add tenderloin, onion and bell pepper; toss to coat well. Let stand 20 minutes.

2. Alternately thread meat and vegetables onto four long skewers. Brush any remaining marinade from dish over meat and vegetables.

3. Grill skewers on covered grill 5 minutes on each side. (Tenderloin will be pink in center and vegetables will be crisp-tender.) Top with thyme.

$1/3$ cup light Caesar salad dressing

3 cloves garlic, minced

1 pound beef tenderloin tips or steaks, cut into $1\frac{1}{2}$-inch chunks

1 small red onion (or $\frac{1}{2}$ medium), cut into $\frac{1}{2}$-inch-thick wedges

1 large red or yellow bell pepper (or $\frac{1}{2}$ of each), cut into 1-inch chunks

2 tablespoons chopped fresh thyme or rosemary

Calories 252, **Total Fat** 12g, **Saturated Fat** 3g, **Cholesterol** 85mg, **Sodium** 313mg, **Carbohydrates** 8g, **Dietary Fiber** 1g, **Protein** 27g
Dietary Exchanges: 3 Meat, 2 Vegetable, $\frac{1}{2}$ Fat

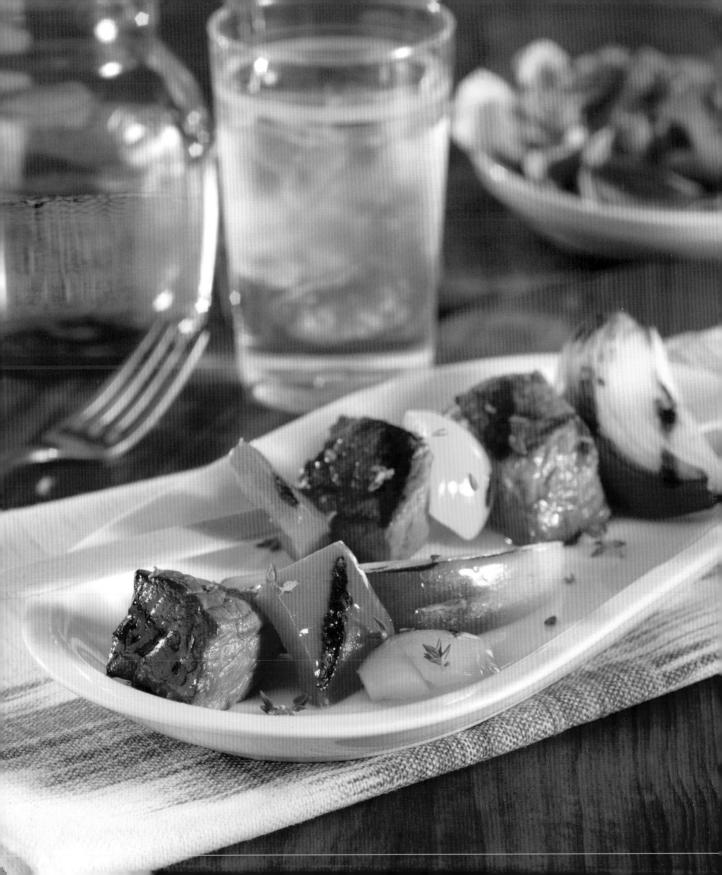

GRILLED TUNA WITH CHICKPEA SALAD
MAKES 4 SERVINGS (3 OUNCES TUNA AND 1/2 CUP SALAD PER SERVING)

1. Combine lime juice, 1 teaspoon mustard, 1 teaspoon oil, 1/4 teaspoon black pepper and 1 tablespoon chives in shallow bowl. Add tuna; turn to coat. Marinate at room temperature 30 minutes.

2. Meanwhile, combine bell pepper, chickpeas, jalapeño pepper and shallot in medium bowl. Stir together remaining 2 teaspoons oil, broth, lemon juice, remaining 2 teaspoons mustard, salt, remaining 1/4 teaspoon black pepper and oregano in small bowl. Pour over chickpea mixture; stir well.

3. Coat grill pan or large skillet with nonstick cooking spray; heat over medium-high heat. Cook tuna 5 minutes per side or until done, but slightly pink in center. (Tuna will continue to cook when removed from heat.)

4. Cut each tuna steak in half. Sprinkle with remaining 1 tablespoon chives. Serve salad on spinach leaves. Garnish with lemon or lime wedges, if desired.

- 2 tablespoons fresh lime juice
- 3 teaspoons Dijon mustard, divided
- 3 teaspoons olive oil, divided
- 1/2 teaspoon black pepper, divided
- 2 tablespoons minced fresh chives, divided
- 2 tuna steaks (6 ounces each), 1 inch thick
- 1 large red bell pepper, diced
- 1 can (about 15 ounces) no-salt-added chickpeas, rinsed and drained
- 1 medium jalapeño pepper,* minced
- 1 large shallot, minced
- 2 tablespoons chicken broth
- 1 teaspoon lemon juice
- 1/4 teaspoon salt
- 1/8 teaspoon dried oregano
- Fresh spinach leaves
- Lemon or lime wedges (optional)

*Jalapeño peppers can sting and irritate the skin, so wear rubber gloves when handling peppers and do not touch your eyes.

Calories 275, **Total Fat** 8g, **Saturated Fat** 2g, **Cholesterol** 32mg, **Sodium** 318mg, **Carbohydrates** 23g, **Dietary Fiber** 1g, **Protein** 26g
Dietary Exchanges: 1 1/2 Bread/Starch, 3 Meat

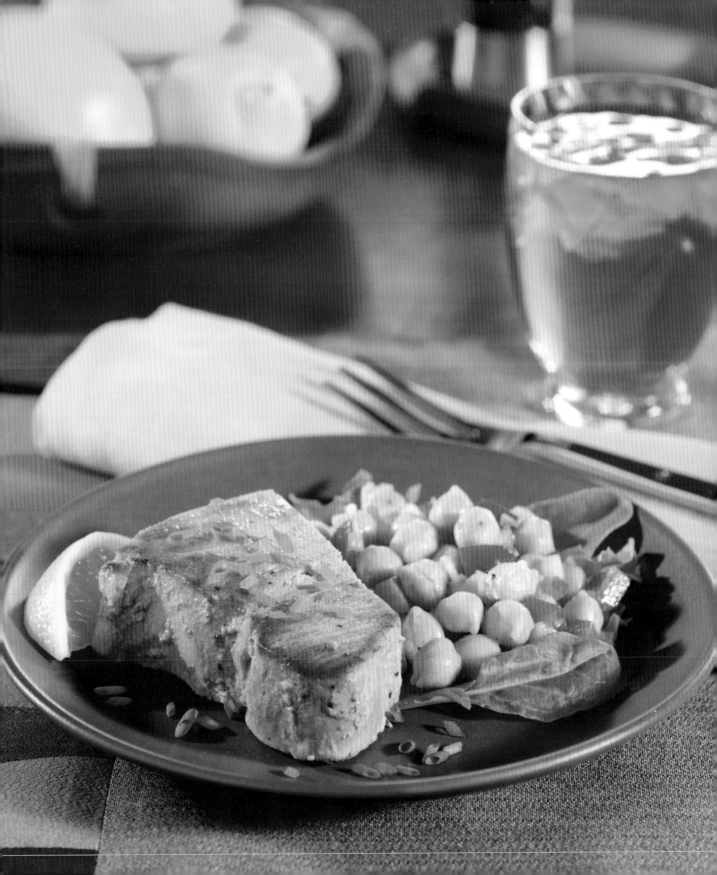

ROASTED TURKEY BREAST WITH APPLE-BALSAMIC GLAZE

MAKES 12 SERVINGS (ABOUT 3 OUNCES TURKEY AND ABOUT 2 TABLESPOONS GLAZE PER SERVING)

1. Preheat oven to 325°F. Combine chili powder, cumin, allspice, ground red pepper and black pepper in small bowl; stir until well blended. Loosen skin on turkey breast by sliding fingertips between skin and meat; do not remove skin. Rub chili mixture on meat of turkey. Coat 13×9-inch baking rack and pan with nonstick cooking spray, place turkey on rack; cook 1 hour 45 minutes or until meat thermometer reaches 165°F.

2. Remove turkey from oven. Place on cutting board; let stand 20 minutes before slicing.

3. Heat oil in large nonstick skillet over medium-high heat, add onion; cook 4 minutes or until onion is soft.

4. Meanwhile, stir together vinegar and cornstarch in small bowl until dissolved. Add cornstarch mixture and remaining ingredients to onion. Bring to a boil over medium-high heat; boil 5 to 6 minutes or until apples are just tender. Remove from heat and let stand, uncovered, 5 minutes to absorb flavors. Serve with sliced turkey.

2 teaspoons chili powder

1 teaspoon ground cumin

1/2 teaspoon ground allspice

1/4 teaspoon ground red pepper

1/2 teaspoon black pepper

1 (6-pound) bone-in turkey breast, thawed, rinsed and patted dry

GLAZE

1 teaspoon canola oil

1/2 cup diced red onion

2 tablespoons balsamic vinegar

1 1/2 teaspoons cornstarch

1 1/2 cups diced (1/4-inch pieces) red apple, unpeeled

1 cup apple cider or apple juice

1 to 2 tablespoons packed sucralose-brown sugar blend

1/2 teaspoon ground cinnamon

1/4 teaspoon salt

Calories 180, **Total Fat** 7g, **Saturated Fat** 0g, **Cholesterol** 20mg, **Sodium** 170 mg, **Carbohydrates** 7g, **Dietary Fiber** 1g, **Protein** 24g
Dietary Exchanges: 3 Meat, 1/2 Fruit

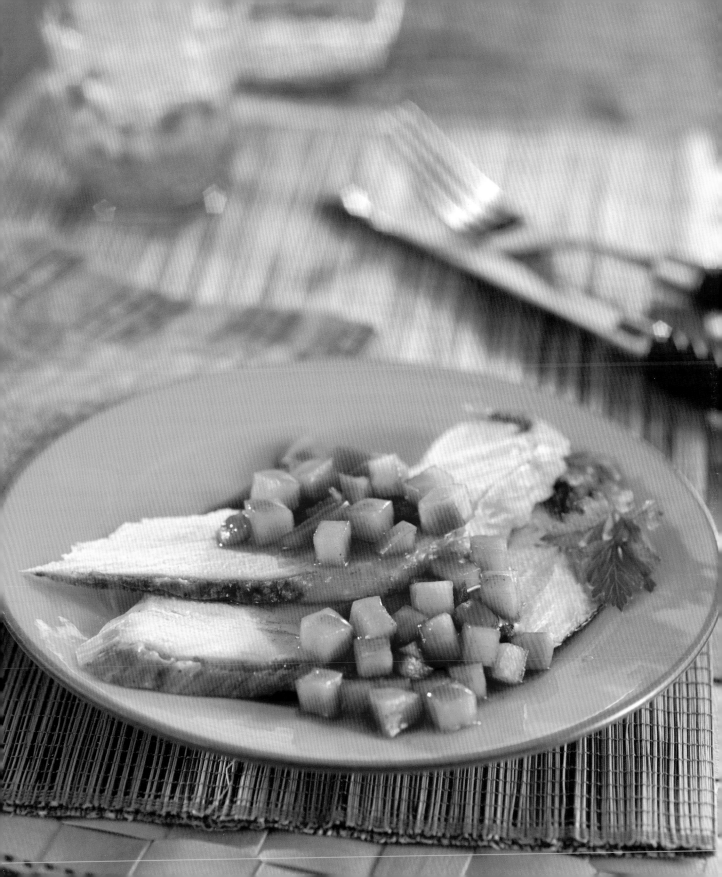

ROASTED SALMON AND ASPARAGUS WITH QUINOA

MAKES 4 SERVINGS

1. Preheat oven to 400°F. Place asparagus in large nonstick roasting pan. Drizzle with 1 teaspoon oil. Roast 10 minutes. Push asparagus to one side of pan. Arrange salmon, skin side down, on other side. Brush with ½ teaspoon oil, sprinkle with ½ teaspoon salt and ⅛ teaspoon pepper. Roast 10 to 13 minutes or until salmon is cooked through. Remove asparagus; cut into bite-size pieces.

2. Meanwhile, place quinoa in fine-mesh strainer; rinse well under cold running water. Bring 1 cup water to a boil in small saucepan; stir in quinoa. Reduce heat to low; cover and simmer 10 to 15 minutes or until quinoa is tender and water is absorbed. Transfer to large bowl.

3. Stir in asparagus, green onion, remaining 1 teaspoon oil, ½ teaspoon salt, ⅛ teaspoon pepper, lemon juice and dill. Transfer to four plates; top with salmon. Garnish with lemon wedges.

1 pound fresh thin asparagus spears

2½ teaspoons olive oil, divided

8 ounces wild-caught salmon fillet

1 teaspoon salt, divided

¼ teaspoon black pepper, divided

½ cup uncooked quinoa

1 cup water

1 green onion, chopped

1 teaspoon lemon juice

½ teaspoon minced fresh dill

4 lemon wedges (optional)

Calories 220, **Total Fat** 8g, **Saturated Fat** 1g, **Cholesterol** 35mg, **Sodium** 620mg, **Carbohydrates** 19g, **Dietary Fiber** 4g, **Protein** 18g
Dietary Exchanges: 1 Bread/Starch, 2 Meat, 1 Vegetable, ½ Fruit

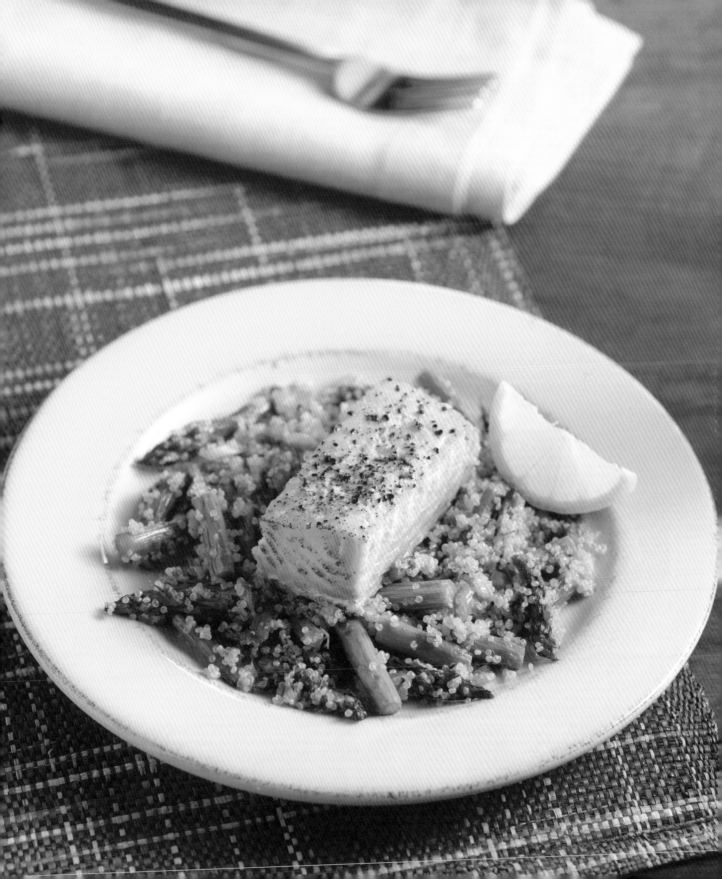

SHRIMP PAD THAI

MAKES 2 TO 4 SERVINGS

1. For sauce, combine ¹/₂ cup cilantro, jalapeño pepper, lime juice, vinegar, peanut butter, water, sugar, soy sauce and red pepper flakes in blender or food processor. Blend until smooth.

2. Cook pasta according to package directions, omitting any salt or fat. Add shrimp during last 3 minutes of cooking; cook until shrimp are opaque and pasta is tender. Add snow peas; drain immediately. Transfer to large bowl. Add sauce; stir until well blended. Sprinkle with green onions and peanuts; toss gently. Garnish with remaining 2 tablespoons cilantro and lime wedges.

¹/₂ cup plus 2 tablespoons chopped fresh cilantro, divided

1 medium jalapeño pepper,* stemmed

2 tablespoons fresh lime juice

2 tablespoons rice vinegar or white vinegar

2 tablespoons unsalted natural peanut butter

2 tablespoons water

1¹/₂ tablespoons sugar

2 teaspoons reduced-sodium soy sauce

¹/₄ teaspoon red pepper flakes

4 ounces uncooked whole grain vermicelli or spaghetti, broken in half

8 ounces raw shrimp, peeled

3 ounces snow peas, cut in half diagonally

¹/₂ cup chopped green onions

2 ounces unsalted peanuts, toasted** and finely chopped

1 medium lime, quartered

*Jalapeño peppers can sting and irritate the skin, so wear rubber gloves when handling peppers and do not touch your eyes.

**To toast peanuts, spread in single layer in heavy skillet. Cook over medium heat 1 to 2 minutes or until nuts are lightly browned, stirring frequently.

Calories 315, **Total Fat** 12g, **Saturated Fat** 2g, **Cholesterol** 71mg, **Sodium** 444mg, **Carbohydrates** 35g, **Dietary Fiber** 6g, **Protein** 18g
Dietary Exchanges: 1 Bread/Starch, 2 Meat, 1 Vegetable, 2¹/₂ Fat

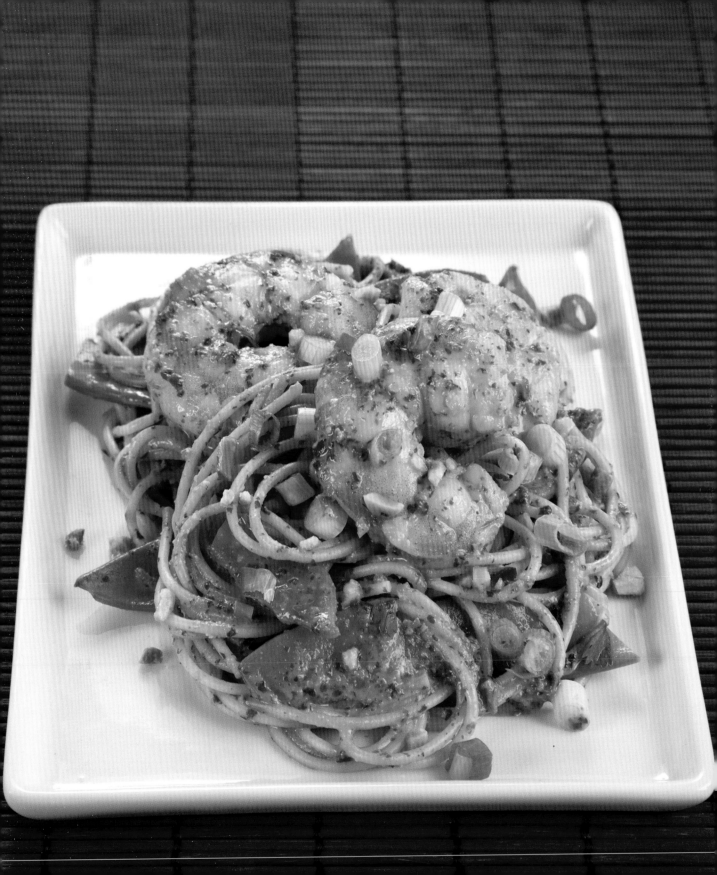

TURKEY-TORTILLA BAKE

MAKES 4 SERVINGS

1. Preheat oven to 400°F. Place tortillas on large baking sheet, overlapping as little as possible. Bake 4 minutes. Turn tortillas; bake 2 minutes or until crisp. Remove to wire rack to cool completely.

2. Heat medium nonstick skillet over medium heat. Add turkey and onion; cook and stir 5 minutes or until turkey is browned and onion is tender. Stir in taco sauce, chiles and corn; mix well. Reduce heat to low; cook 5 minutes.

3. Break up 3 tortillas; arrange pieces on bottom of 1½-quart casserole. Spoon half of turkey mixture over tortillas; sprinkle with half of cheese. Repeat layers.

4. Bake 10 minutes or until cheese is melted and casserole is heated through. Break remaining 3 tortillas into pieces and sprinkle over casserole. Serve with sour cream, if desired.

9 (6-inch) corn tortillas

½ pound 93% lean ground turkey

½ cup chopped onion

¾ cup taco sauce

1 can (4 ounces) chopped mild green chiles, drained

½ cup frozen corn, thawed and drained

½ cup (2 ounces) shredded reduced-fat Cheddar cheese

Fat-free sour cream (optional)

Calories 279, **Total Fat** 8g, **Saturated Fat** 2g, **Cholesterol** 26mg, **Sodium** 666mg, **Carbohydrates** 38g, **Dietary Fiber** 1g, **Protein** 17g
Dietary Exchanges: 2½ Bread/Starch, 1 Meat, 1 Fat

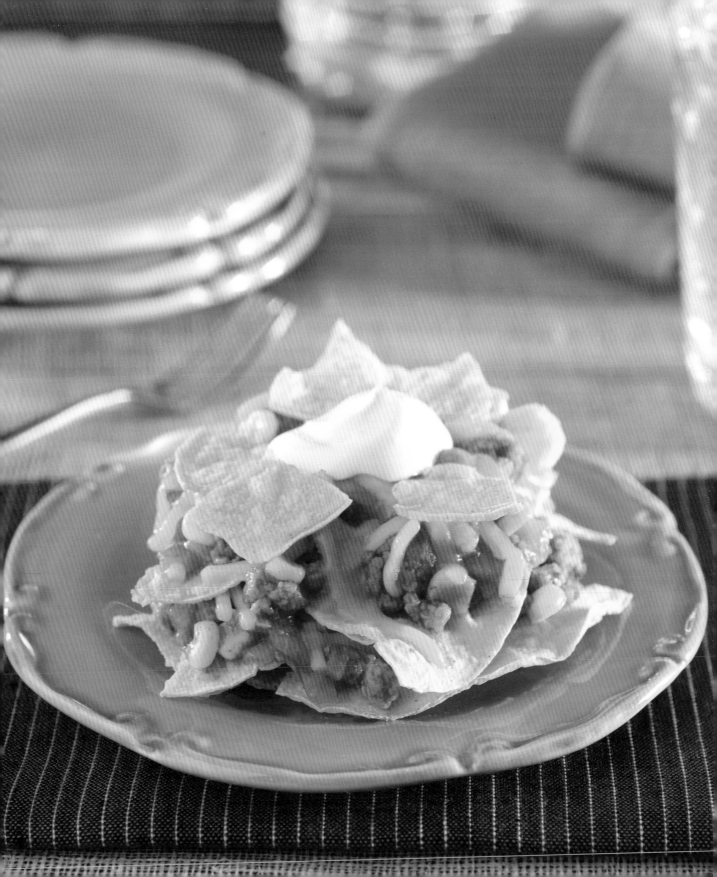

BEEF & ARTICHOKE CASSEROLE

MAKES 4 SERVINGS

1. Preheat oven to 400°F. Spray 1-quart casserole with nonstick cooking spray.

2. Brown beef in medium skillet over medium-high heat 6 to 8 minutes, stirring to break up meat. Drain fat. Add mushrooms, onion and garlic; cook and stir 5 minutes or until tender.

3. Combine ground beef mixture, artichokes, bread crumbs, Parmesan cheese, rosemary and marjoram; gently mix. Season with salt and pepper, if desired.

4. Beat egg whites in medium bowl with electric mixer at high speed until stiff peaks form; fold into ground beef mixture. Spoon into prepared casserole.

5. Bake 20 minutes or until edges are lightly browned.

¾ pound 95% lean ground beef

½ cup sliced mushrooms

¼ cup chopped onion

1 clove garlic, minced

1 can (14 ounces) artichoke hearts, drained and chopped

½ cup dry bread crumbs

¼ cup (1 ounce) grated Parmesan cheese

1 tablespoon chopped fresh rosemary leaves *or* 1 teaspoon dried rosemary

1½ teaspoons chopped fresh marjoram *or* ½ teaspoon dried marjoram

Salt and black pepper (optional)

3 egg whites

Calories 260, **Total Fat** 7g, **Saturated Fat** 3g, **Cholesterol** 55mg, **Sodium** 330mg, **Carbohydrates** 24g, **Dietary Fiber** 9g, **Protein** 28g
Dietary Exchanges: ½ Bread/Starch, 3 Meat, 2½ Vegetable

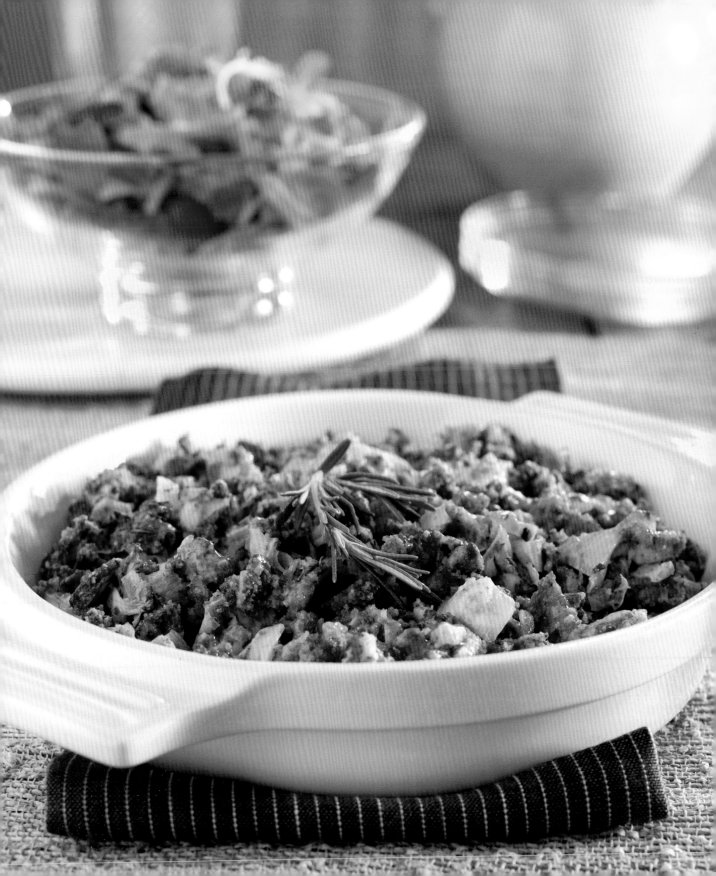

SAUCY TOMATO-PORK SKILLET

MAKES 4 SERVINGS

1. Prepare rice according to package directions; set aside.

2. Combine tomato juice, soy sauce, cornstarch and paprika in small bowl, stirring until cornstarch dissolves. Set aside.

3. Slice pork across grain into ¼-inch slices; place in medium bowl. Sprinkle pork with garlic salt and red pepper flakes; mix well.

4. Cook bacon in medium skillet over medium-high heat. Remove bacon from skillet using slotted spoon; set aside. Add pork, tomatoes and green onions to skillet; stir-fry over medium-high heat 3 minutes or until pork is barely pink in center. Stir in tomato juice mixture; cook, stirring constantly, 1 minute or until sauce thickens slightly. Remove from heat; stir in bacon.

5. Serve pork mixture over rice.

1 cup uncooked instant white rice

⅔ cup reduced-sodium tomato juice

2 tablespoons reduced-sodium soy sauce

1 tablespoon cornstarch

¼ teaspoon paprika

3 boneless pork chops, cut ¾ inch thick (about ¾ pound)

¼ teaspoon garlic salt

⅛ teaspoon red pepper flakes

2 slices uncooked bacon, chopped

3 medium tomatoes, chopped

2 green onions with tops, sliced diagonally

Calories 307, **Total Fat** 10g, **Saturated Fat** 3g, **Cholesterol** 62mg, **Sodium** 492mg, **Carbohydrates** 26g, **Dietary Fiber** 1g, **Protein** 23g
Dietary Exchanges: 1½ Bread/Starch, 2 Meat, 1 Vegetable, 1 Fat

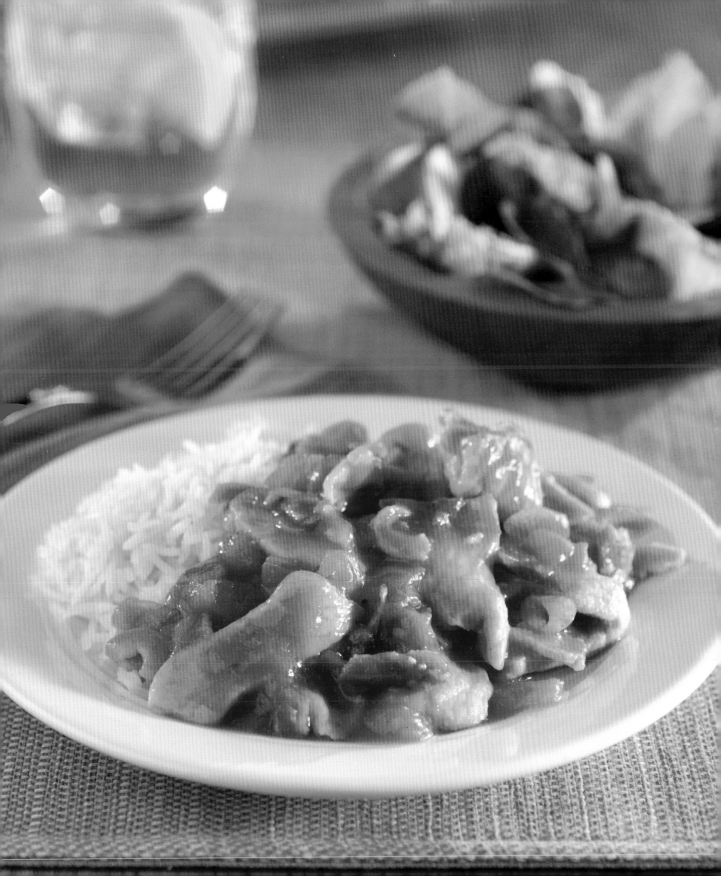

ROASTED SALMON WITH STRAWBERRY-ORANGE SALSA

MAKES 4 SERVINGS

1. Preheat oven to 400°F.

2. Line baking sheet with foil; spray with nonstick cooking spray. Place salmon on prepared baking sheet; sprinkle with cumin, thyme, salt and black pepper. Bake 12 to 14 minutes or until salmon begins to flake when tested with fork.

3. Meanwhile, grate orange peel to measure 1/2 teaspoon; place in medium bowl. Peel and section orange; coarsely chop orange sections. Add orange sections, strawberries, poblano pepper, cilantro and ginger to bowl; mix well. Serve salmon with salsa.

- 4 **salmon fillets (about 1/4 pound each), skin removed**
- 1/2 **teaspoon ground cumin**
- 1/2 **teaspoon dried thyme**
- 1/4 **teaspoon salt**
- 1/4 **teaspoon black pepper**
- 1 **medium orange**
- 1 **cup diced fresh strawberries**
- 1/4 **cup finely chopped poblano pepper* or green bell pepper**
- 2 **tablespoons finely chopped fresh cilantro**
- 1/2 **teaspoon grated fresh ginger**

*Poblano peppers can sting and irritate the skin, so wear rubber gloves when handling peppers and do not touch your eyes.

Calories 270, **Total Fat** 15g, **Saturated Fat** 4g, **Cholesterol** 60mg, **Sodium** 220mg, **Carbohydrates** 9g, **Dietary Fiber** 2g, **Protein** 24g
Dietary Exchanges: 3 Meat, 1/2 Fruit, 1 Fat

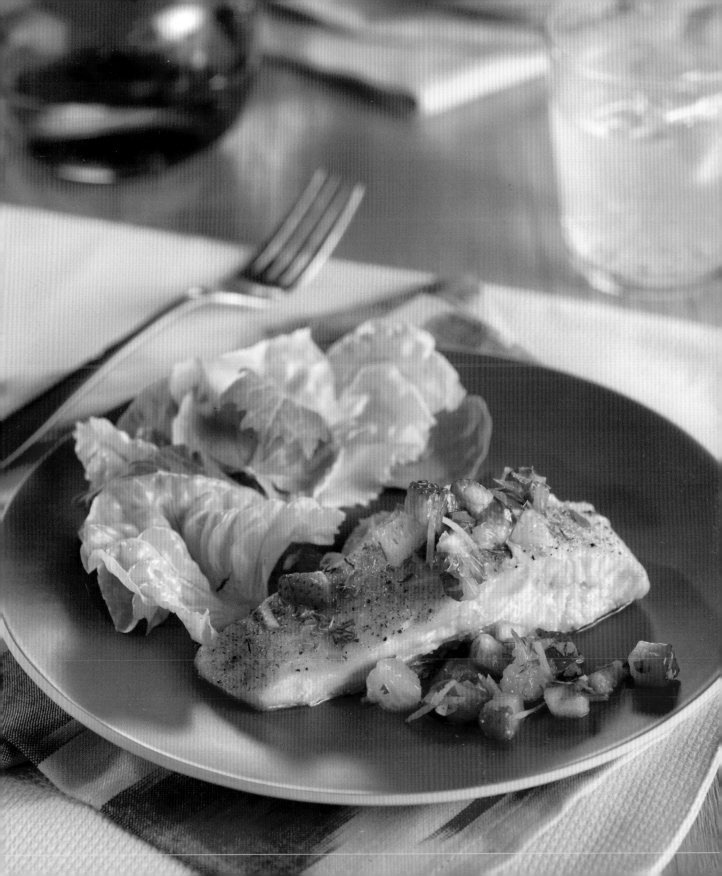

ROASTED ALMOND TILAPIA
MAKES 2 SERVINGS

1. Preheat oven to 450°F. Place fish on small baking sheet; season with salt. Spread mustard over fish. Combine bread crumbs and almonds in small bowl; sprinkle over fish. Press lightly to adhere. Sprinkle with paprika, if desired.

2. Bake 8 to 10 minutes or until fish is opaque in center and begins to flake when tested with fork. Serve with lemon wedges, if desired.

2 tilapia or Boston scrod fillets (6 ounces each)

¼ teaspoon salt

1 tablespoon prepared mustard

¼ cup whole wheat bread crumbs

2 tablespoons chopped almonds

Paprika (optional)

Lemon wedges (optional)

Calories 272, **Total Fat** 6g, **Saturated Fat** 2g, **Cholesterol** 84mg, **Sodium** 464mg, **Carbohydrates** 17g, **Dietary Fiber** 1g, **Protein** 37g
Dietary Exchanges: 1 Bread/Starch, 4 Meat

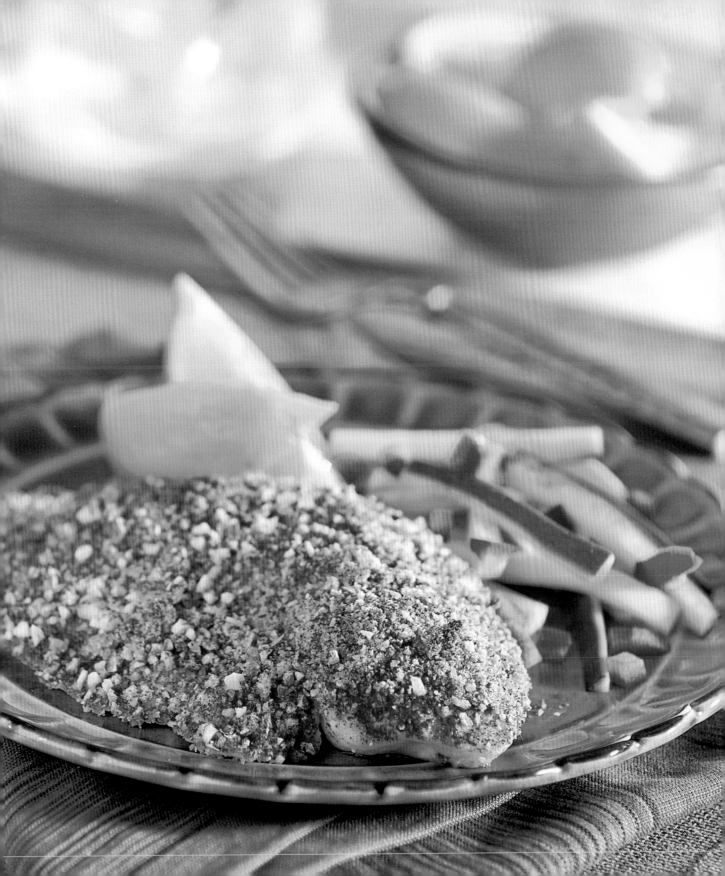

SPICY LEMONY ALMOND CHICKEN

MAKES 4 SERVINGS

1. Combine paprika, pepper and salt in small bowl; sprinkle evenly over both sides of chicken.

2. Coat large nonstick skillet with nonstick cooking spray. Heat over medium-high heat; add chicken. Cook 3 to 4 minutes on each side or until no longer pink in center; set aside on serving platter. Sprinkle with almonds; cover to keep warm.

3. Add water, lemon juice, margarine and Worcestershire sauce to skillet; stir until pan sauces are reduced to $1/4$ cup, scraping bottom and side of skillet. Remove from heat, stir in lemon peel; spoon evenly over chicken.

TIP: To pound chicken, place between two pieces of plastic wrap. Starting in the center, pound chicken with a meat mallet to reach an even thickness.

$1/2$ teaspoon paprika

$1/2$ teaspoon black pepper

$1/4$ teaspoon salt

4 boneless skinless chicken breasts (about 1 pound total), flattened to $1/4$-inch thickness

1 ounce slivered almonds, toasted

$1/4$ cup water

2 tablespoons lemon juice

2 tablespoons reduced-fat margarine

2 teaspoons Worcestershire sauce

$1/2$ teaspoon grated lemon peel

Calories 193, **Total Fat** 7g, **Saturated Fat** 1g, **Cholesterol** 66mg, **Sodium** 257mg, **Carbohydrates** 3g, **Dietary Fiber** 1g, **Protein** 28g
Dietary Exchanges: 3 Meat

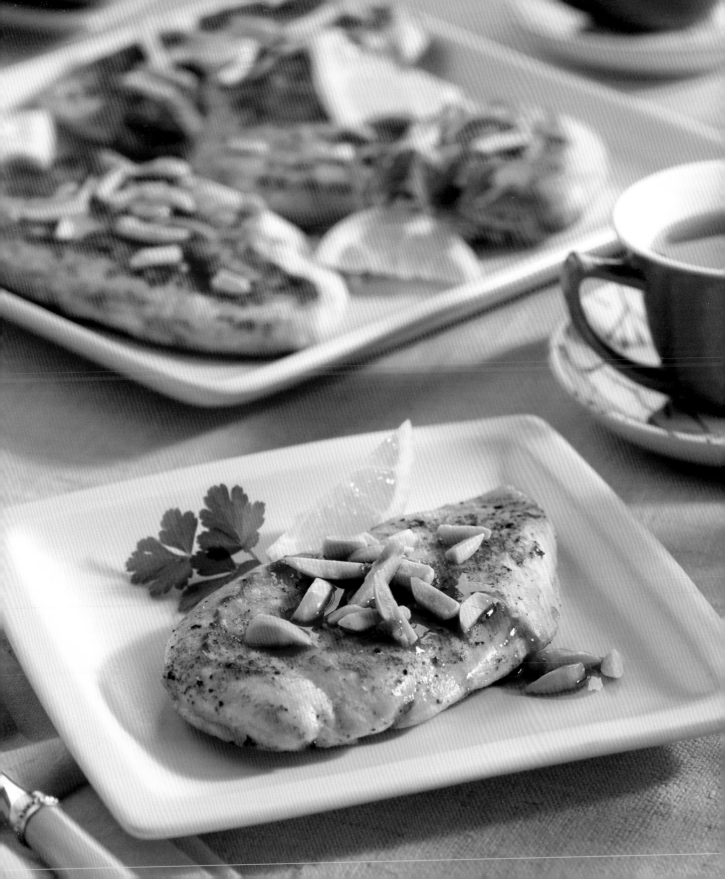

MEXICAN BLACK BEAN CASSEROLE

MAKES 4 SERVINGS

1. Heat oven to 375°F. Place beans in large bowl; partially mash with potato masher or bottom of heavy glass. Add chicken, green onions, salsa, tomatoes and cumin; mix well. Spoon 1¹/₃ cups mixture into 9-inch round glass baking dish; top with ¹/₂ cup cheese. Arrange 1 tortilla over mixture, tearing to fit size of dish. Repeat layering with 1¹/₃ cups bean mixture, remaining tortilla and remaining bean mixture. Cover dish with foil; bake 30 minutes or until heated through.

2. Remove from oven. Uncover; top with remaining ¹/₄ cup cheese. Return to oven; continue to bake 5 minutes or until cheese is melted. Remove from oven; top with cilantro.

1 can (about 15 ounces) no-salt-added black beans, rinsed and drained

1¹/₂ cups (6 ounces) shredded cooked chicken

4 large green onions, sliced

1 cup salsa

³/₄ cup diced tomatoes

2 teaspoons ground cumin

³/₄ cup (3 ounces) shredded reduced-fat Mexican cheese blend, divided

2 (9-inch) whole wheat flour tortillas, divided

¹/₄ cup chopped fresh cilantro

Calories 290, **Total Fat** 7g, **Saturated Fat** 3g, **Cholesterol** 50mg, **Sodium** 600mg, **Carbohydrates** 32g, **Dietary Fiber** 11g, **Protein** 29g
Dietary Exchanges: 1¹/₂ Bread/Starch, 3 Meat, 1 Vegetable

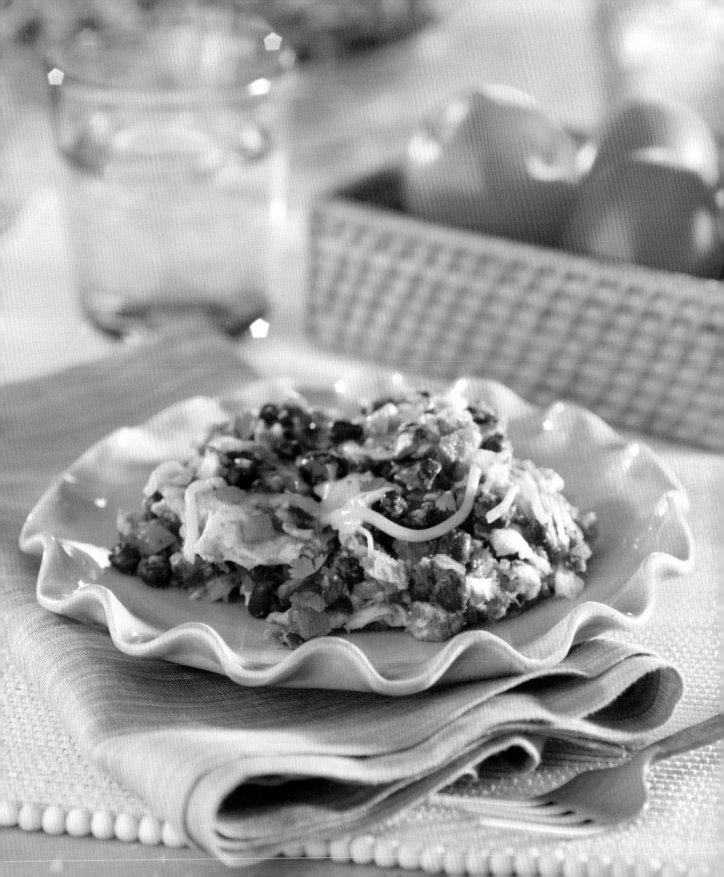

PASTA WITH TUNA, GREEN BEANS & TOMATOES

MAKES 6 SERVINGS

1. Cook pasta according to package directions, omitting salt and fat. Add green beans during last 7 minutes of cooking time (allow water to return to a boil before resuming timing). Drain and keep warm.

2. Meanwhile, heat 1 teaspoon oil in large skillet over medium heat. Add green onions and garlic; cook and stir 2 minutes. Add tomatoes, salt, Italian seasoning and pepper; cook and stir 4 to 5 minutes. Add pasta mixture, tuna and remaining 2 teaspoons oil; mix gently. Garnish with parsley. Serve immediately.

8 ounces uncooked whole wheat penne, rigatoni or fusilli pasta

1½ cups frozen cut green beans

3 teaspoons olive oil, divided

3 green onions, sliced

1 clove garlic, minced

1 can (about 14 ounces) diced Italian-style tomatoes, drained *or* 2 large tomatoes, chopped (about 2 cups)

½ teaspoon salt

½ teaspoon Italian seasoning

¼ teaspoon black pepper

1 can (12 ounces) solid albacore tuna packed in water, drained and flaked

Chopped fresh parsley (optional)

Calories 228, **Total Fat** 4g, **Saturated Fat** 1g, **Cholesterol** 14mg, **Sodium** 345mg, **Carbohydrates** 34g, **Dietary Fiber** 3g, **Protein** 15g
Dietary Exchanges: 2 Bread/Starch, 3 Meat, 1 Vegetable

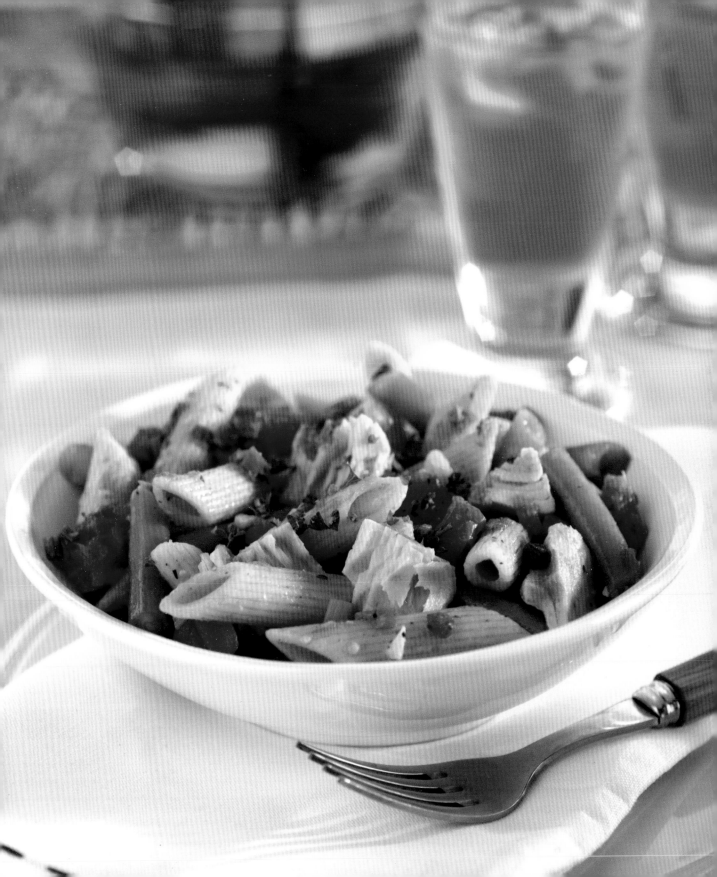

ORANGE CHICKEN

MAKES 4 SERVINGS

1. Combine broth mixture and rice in large saucepan; bring to a boil over high heat. Reduce heat to low; simmer, partially covered, 45 to 55 minutes or until rice is tender. Drain excess liquid; keep warm.

2. Blend orange juice, teriyaki sauce, cornstarch, honey and garlic in small bowl until smooth.

3. Spray large nonstick skillet with nonstick cooking spray; heat over high heat. Add chicken; stir-fry 4 minutes or until chicken is cooked through. Stir orange juice mixture and currants into skillet; bring to a boil. Boil, uncovered, 3 minutes. Add snow peas, orange segments and 1½ teaspoons orange peel. Cook and stir 2 minutes or until heated through. Stir in green onions and cilantro. Spoon over rice. Sprinkle with remaining 1½ teaspoons orange peel.

1 can (about 14 ounces) fat-free reduced-sodium chicken broth, plus water to measure 3 cups

¾ cup uncooked wild rice, rinsed

1 cup orange juice

2 tablespoons reduced-sodium teriyaki sauce

1 teaspoon cornstarch

1 teaspoon honey

2 cloves garlic, minced

¾ pound boneless skinless chicken thighs, cut into thin strips

¼ cup dried currants

8 ounces (2½ to 3 cups) fresh snow peas or 1 package (8 ounces) frozen snow peas, thawed

1 orange, peeled and separated into segments

3 teaspoons grated orange peel, divided

3 green onions, thinly sliced

⅓ cup chopped fresh cilantro

Calories 336, **Total Fat** 3g, **Saturated Fat** 1g, **Cholesterol** 52mg, **Sodium** 343mg, **Carbohydrates** 49g, **Dietary Fiber** 5g, **Protein** 29g
Dietary Exchanges: 3 Bread/Starch, 2 Meat

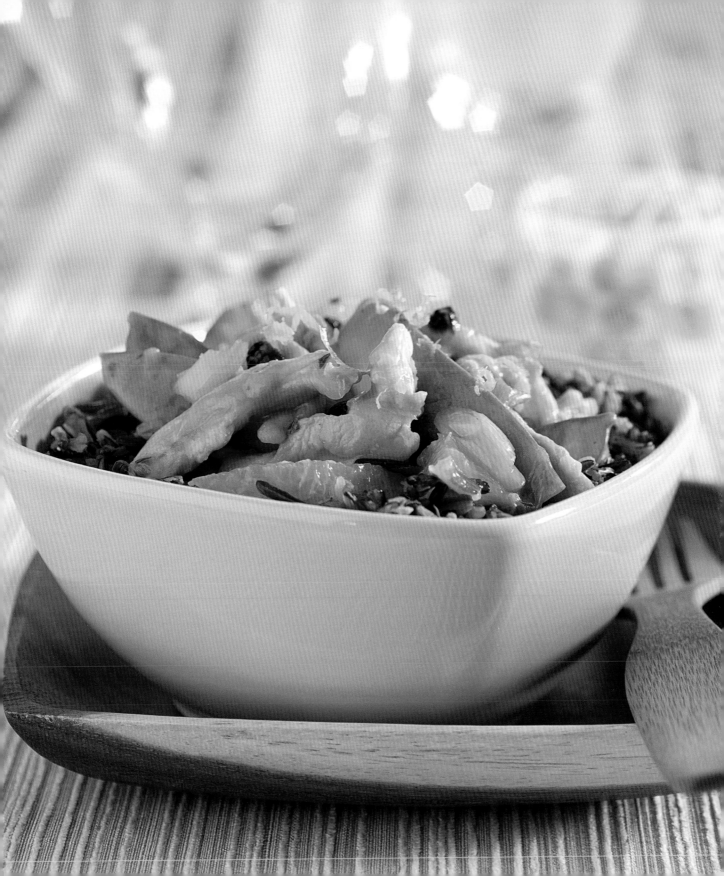

APPLE-CHERRY GLAZED PORK CHOPS

MAKES 2 SERVINGS

1. Combine thyme, salt and pepper in small bowl. Rub onto both sides of pork chops.

2. Spray large skillet with nonstick cooking spray; heat over medium heat. Add pork chops; cook 3 to 5 minutes or until barely pink in center, turning once. Remove to plate; keep warm.

3. Add apple juice, apple slices, green onion and cherries to same skillet. Simmer 2 to 3 minutes or until apple and onion are tender.

4. Stir cornstarch into water in small bowl until smooth; stir into skillet. Bring to a boil; cook and stir until thickened. Spoon apple mixture over pork chops.

$1/4$ to $1/2$ teaspoon dried thyme

$1/8$ teaspoon salt

$1/8$ teaspoon black pepper

2 boneless pork loin chops (3 ounces each), trimmed of fat

$2/3$ cup unsweetened apple juice

$1/2$ small apple, sliced

2 tablespoons sliced green onion

2 tablespoons dried tart cherries

1 teaspoon cornstarch

1 tablespoon water

Calories 243, **Total Fat** 8g, **Saturated Fat** 3g, **Cholesterol** 40mg, **Sodium** 191mg, **Carbohydrates** 23g, **Dietary Fiber** 1g, **Protein** 19g
Dietary Exchanges: 2 Meat, $1^{1}/2$ Fruit, 1 Fat

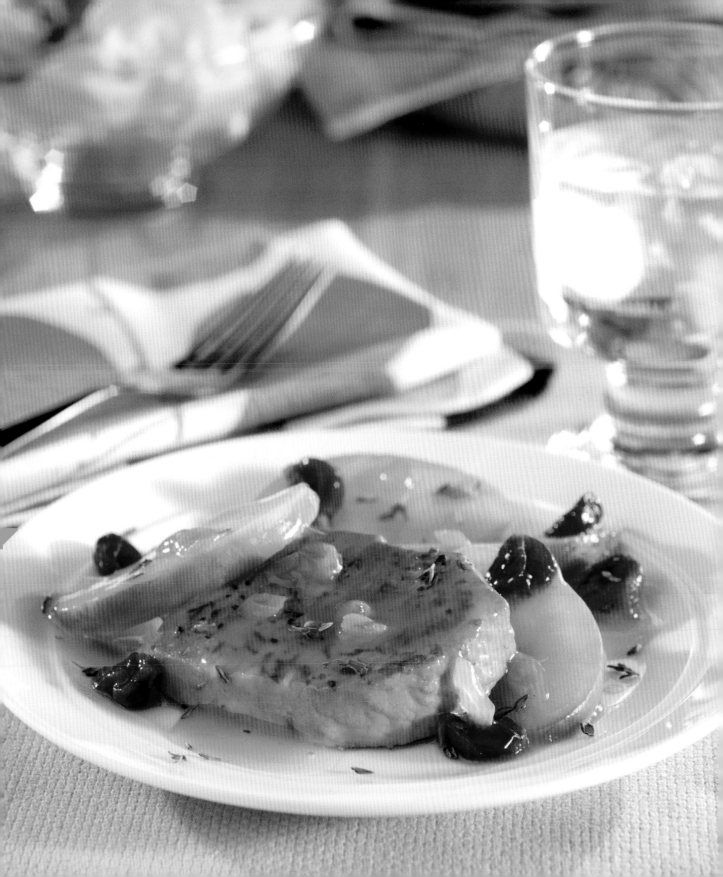

CHICKEN & WILD RICE SKILLET DINNER

MAKES 1 SERVING

1. Melt margarine in small skillet over medium-high heat. Add chicken; cook and stir 3 to 5 minutes or until cooked through.

2. Meanwhile, measure 1/4 cup of the rice and 1 tablespoon plus 1/2 teaspoon of the seasoning mix. Reserve remaining rice and seasoning mix for another use.

3. Add rice, seasoning mix, water and apricots to skillet; mix well. Bring to a boil. Cover and reduce heat to low; simmer 25 minutes or until liquid is absorbed and rice is tender.

1 teaspoon reduced-fat margarine

2 ounces boneless skinless chicken breast, cut into strips (about 1/2 chicken breast)

1 package (about 5 ounces) long grain and wild rice mix with seasoning

1/2 cup water

3 dried apricots, cut up

Calories 314, **Total Fat** 5g, **Saturated Fat** 1g, **Cholesterol** 52mg, **Sodium** 669mg, **Carbohydrates** 44g, **Dietary Fiber** 3g, **Protein** 24g
Dietary Exchanges: 3 Bread/Starch, 2 Meat, 1/2 Fat

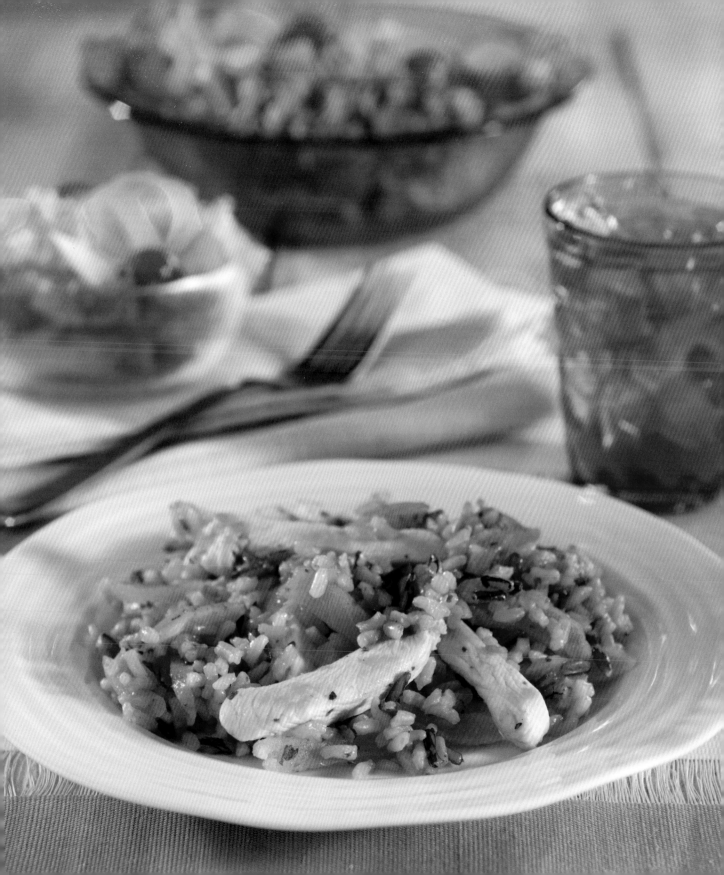

PORK TENDERLOIN WITH CABBAGE

MAKES 6 SERVINGS

1. Preheat oven to 450°F. Pour broth into shallow nonstick roasting pan; heat on stovetop over medium heat. Add cabbage, onion and garlic; cook and stir 2 to 3 minutes or until cabbage wilts.

2. Add pork to roasting pan. (If using two small tenderloins, place side-by-side.) Transfer pan to oven; roast 10 minutes.

3. Meanwhile, combine apple juice concentrate, mustard and Worcestershire sauce in small bowl. Pour half of mixture over pork. Roast 10 minutes.

4. Baste pork with half of remaining apple juice mixture; stir remaining half into cabbage. Roast 15 to 20 minutes or until meat thermometer inserted in center of pork registers 160°F. Let stand 5 minutes. Slice pork and serve with cabbage and pan juices.

¼ cup chicken broth *or* water

3 cups shredded red cabbage

¼ cup chopped onion

1 clove garlic, minced

1½ pounds pork tenderloin

¾ cup apple juice concentrate

3 tablespoons honey mustard

1½ tablespoons Worcestershire sauce

Calories 227, **Total Fat** 4g, **Saturated Fat** 1g, **Cholesterol** 66mg, **Sodium** 145mg, **Carbohydrates** 21g, **Dietary Fiber** 1g, **Protein** 24g
Dietary Exchanges: 3 Meat, 1 Vegetable, ½ Fruit

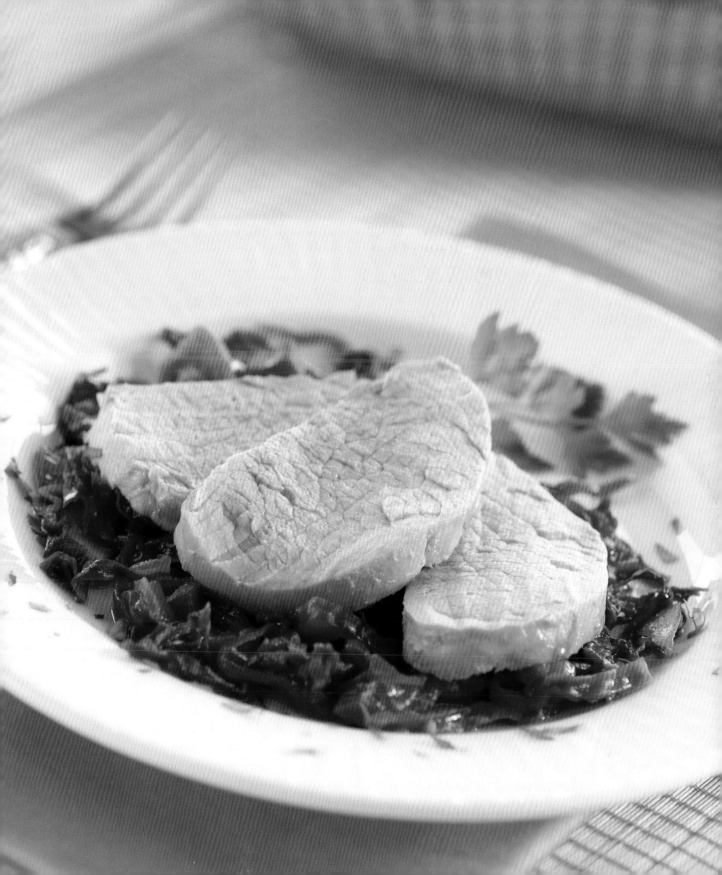

STIR-FRIED BEEF & SPINACH

MAKES 2 SERVINGS

1. Spray large skillet or wok with nonstick cooking spray; heat over high heat. Add spinach; stir-fry 1 minute or until wilted. Transfer spinach to serving platter. Sprinkle with salt; keep warm.

2. Spray same skillet with cooking spray; heat over high heat. Add beef; stir-fry 2 minutes or until barely pink. Add stir-fry sauce, sugar, curry powder and ginger; cook and stir $1\frac{1}{2}$ minutes or until sauce thickens. Serve with spinach.

1 package (6 ounces) fresh spinach, stemmed and torn

$\frac{1}{8}$ teaspoon salt

8 ounces boneless beef top sirloin steak, thinly sliced

$\frac{1}{4}$ cup stir-fry sauce

1 teaspoon sugar

$\frac{1}{2}$ teaspoon curry powder

$\frac{1}{4}$ teaspoon ground ginger

Calories 196, **Total Fat** 7g, **Saturated Fat** 2g, **Cholesterol** 69mg, **Sodium** 799mg, **Carbohydrates** 6g, **Dietary Fiber** 8g, **Protein** 28g
Dietary Exchanges: 3 Meat, 1 Vegetable

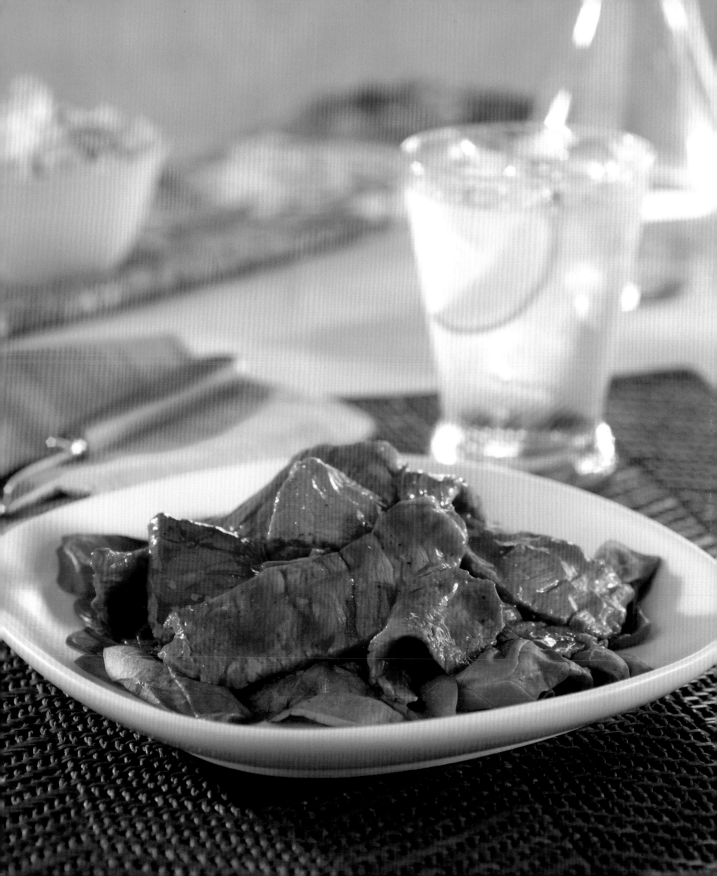

CHICKEN PICCATA
MAKES 4 SERVINGS

1. Combine flour, salt and pepper in shallow dish. Reserve 1 tablespoon flour mixture.

2. Pound chicken between waxed paper to $1/2$-inch thickness with flat side of meat mallet or rolling pin. Coat chicken with remaining flour mixture, shaking off excess.

3. Heat oil and butter in large nonstick skillet over medium heat. Add chicken; cook 4 to 5 minutes per side or until no longer pink in center. Transfer to serving platter; cover loosely with foil.

4. Add garlic to same skillet; cook and stir 1 minute. Add reserved flour mixture; cook and stir 1 minute. Add broth and lemon juice; cook 2 minutes or until thickened, stirring frequently. Stir in parsley and capers; spoon sauce over chicken.

3 tablespoons all-purpose flour

$1/2$ teaspoon salt

$1/4$ teaspoon black pepper

4 boneless skinless chicken breasts (4 ounces each)

2 teaspoons olive oil

1 teaspoon butter

2 cloves garlic, minced

$3/4$ cup fat-free reduced-sodium chicken broth

1 tablespoon fresh lemon juice

2 tablespoons chopped fresh Italian parsley

1 tablespoon capers, drained

Calories 194, **Total Fat** 6g, **Saturated Fat** 2g, **Cholesterol** 71mg, **Sodium** 473mg, **Carbohydrates** 5g, **Dietary Fiber** 1g, **Protein** 27g
Dietary Exchanges: $1/2$ Bread/Starch, 3 Meat

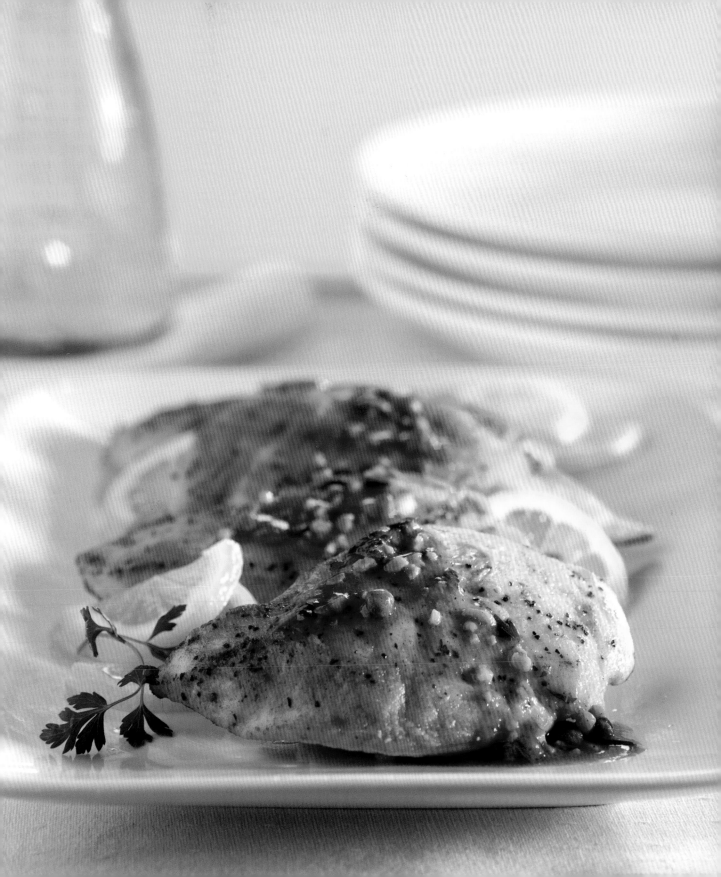

ROAST DILL SCROD WITH ASPARAGUS

MAKES 4 SERVINGS

1. Preheat oven to 425°F.

2. Place asparagus in 13×9-inch baking dish; drizzle with oil. Roll asparagus to coat lightly with oil; push to edges of dish, stacking asparagus into two layers.

3. Arrange fish fillets in center of dish; drizzle with lemon juice. Combine dill weed, salt and pepper in small bowl; sprinkle over fish and asparagus. Sprinkle with paprika, if desired.

4. Roast 15 to 17 minutes or until asparagus is crisp-tender and fish is opaque in center and begins to flake when tested with fork.

1 bunch (12 ounces) asparagus spears, ends trimmed

1 teaspoon olive oil

4 scrod or cod fillets (about 5 ounces each)

1 tablespoon lemon juice

1 teaspoon dried dill weed

½ teaspoon salt

¼ teaspoon black pepper

Paprika (optional)

Calories 147, **Total Fat** 2g, **Saturated Fat** 1g, **Cholesterol** 61mg, **Sodium** 379mg, **Carbohydrates** 4g, **Dietary Fiber** 2g, **Protein** 27g
Dietary Exchanges: 3 Meat, 1 Vegetable

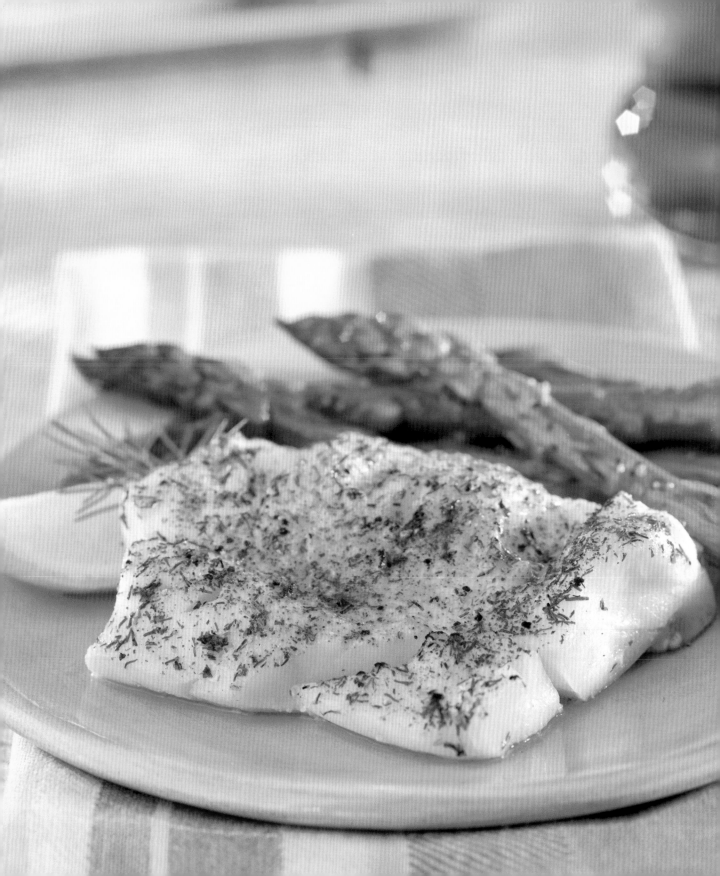

PAN-SEARED HALIBUT STEAKS WITH AVOCADO SALSA

MAKES 4 SERVINGS

1. Combine 2 tablespoons salsa and 1/4 teaspoon salt in small bowl; spread over both sides of halibut.

2. Heat large nonstick skillet over medium heat until hot. Add halibut; cook 4 to 5 minutes per side or until fish is opaque in center.

3. Meanwhile, combine remaining 2 tablespoons salsa, 1/4 teaspoon salt, tomato, avocado and cilantro, if desired, in small bowl. Mix well and spoon over cooked fish. Garnish with lime wedges.

4 **tablespoons chipotle salsa, divided**

1/2 **teaspoon salt, divided**

4 **small (4 to 5 ounces) *or* 2 large (8 to 10 ounces) halibut steaks, cut 3/4 inch thick**

1/2 **cup diced tomato**

1/2 **ripe avocado, diced**

2 **tablespoons chopped fresh cilantro (optional)**

Lime wedges (optional)

Calories 169, **Total Fat** 7g, **Saturated Fat** 1g, **Cholesterol** 36mg, **Sodium** 476mg, **Carbohydrates** 2g, **Dietary Fiber** 4g, **Protein** 25g
Dietary Exchanges: 3 Meat

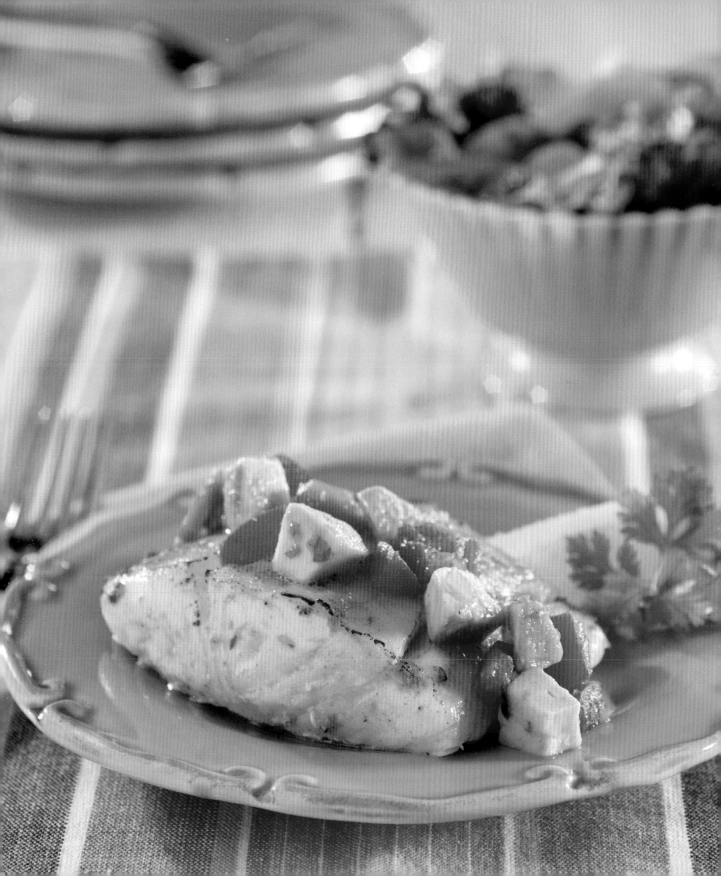

THAI GRILLED CHICKEN

MAKES 4 SERVINGS

1. Prepare grill for direct cooking over medium heat. Place chicken in shallow baking dish. Combine soy sauce, garlic and red pepper flakes in small bowl. Pour over chicken, turning to coat. Let stand 10 minutes.

2. Meanwhile, combine honey and lime juice in small bowl; blend well. Set aside.

3. Place chicken on grid; brush with marinade. Discard remaining marinade. Grill, covered, 5 minutes. Brush both sides of chicken with honey mixture. Grill 5 minutes more or until chicken is no longer pink in center.

SERVING SUGGESTION: Serve with steamed white rice, Oriental vegetables and grilled fruit salad.

- 4 boneless skinless chicken breasts (about 1¼ pounds)
- ¼ cup low-sodium soy sauce
- 2 teaspoons minced garlic
- ½ teaspoon red pepper flakes
- 2 tablespoons honey
- 1 tablespoon fresh lime juice

Calories 140, **Total Fat** 1g, **Saturated Fat** 1g, **Cholesterol** 53mg, **Sodium** 349mg, **Carbohydrates** 10g, **Dietary Fiber** 1g, **Protein** 22g
Dietary Exchanges: 3 Meat, 1 Fruit

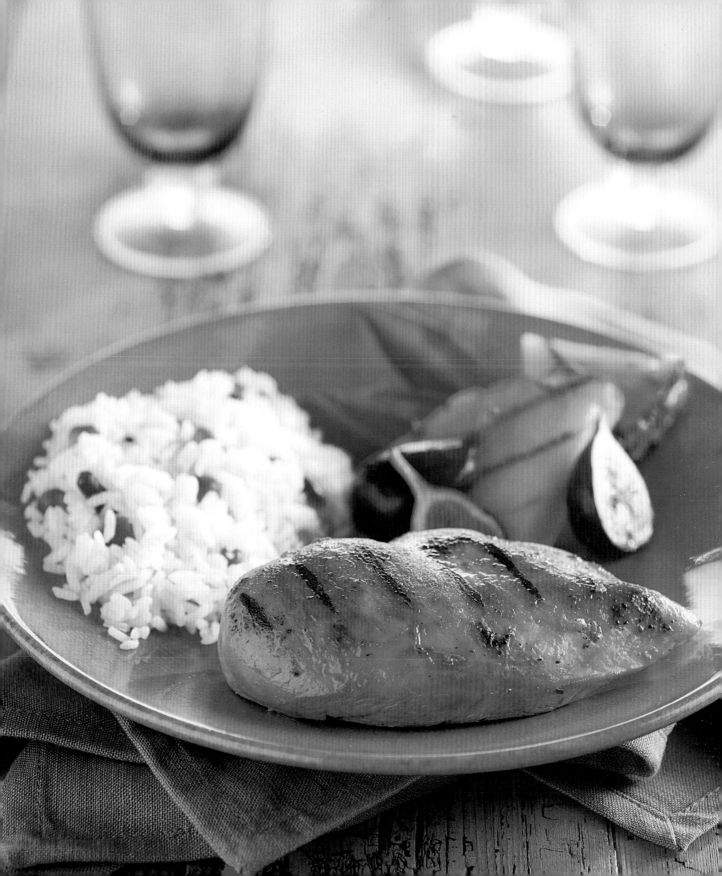

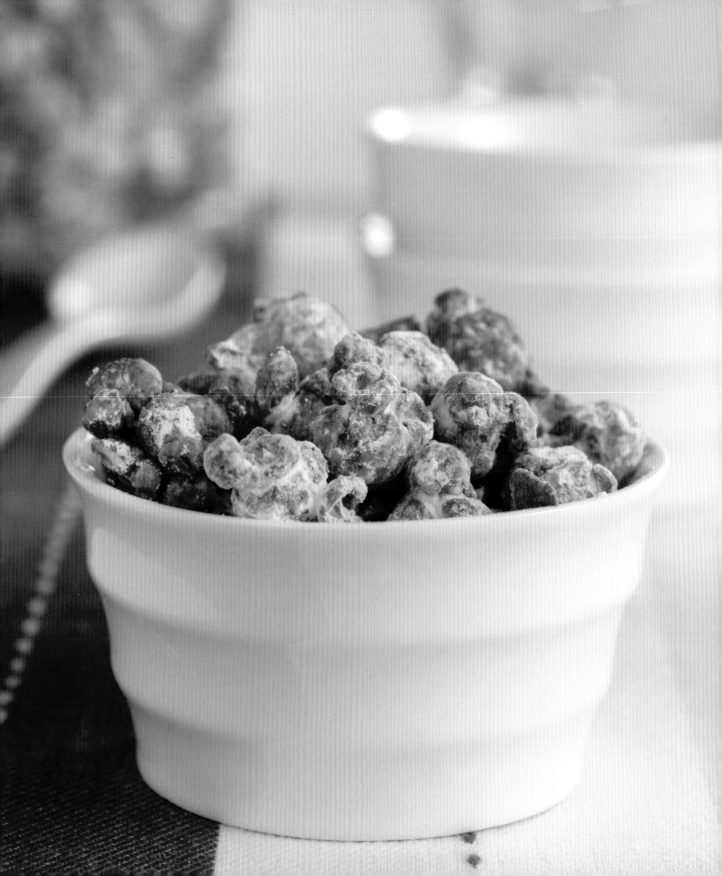

SIMPLE SNACKS

CHOCO-PEANUT BUTTER POPCORN

MAKES 6 SERVINGS

MICROWAVE DIRECTIONS

1. Microwave chocolate chips, peanut butter and butter in medium microwavable bowl on HIGH 30 seconds; stir. Microwave 30 seconds or until melted and smooth. Pour mixture over popcorn in large bowl, stirring until evenly coated. Transfer to 1-gallon resealable food storage bag.

2. Add powdered sugar to bag; seal bag. Shake until well coated. Spread onto waxed paper to cool. Store leftovers in airtight container in refrigerator.

$1/3$ cup semisweet chocolate chips

3 tablespoons natural creamy peanut butter

1 tablespoon trans fat-free butter

4 cups air-popped popcorn

$1/2$ cup powdered sugar

Calories 161, **Total Fat** 9g, **Saturated Fat** 3g, **Cholesterol** 5mg, **Sodium** 19mg, **Carbohydrates** 20g, **Dietary Fiber** 2g, **Protein** 3g
Dietary Exchanges: 1 Bread/Starch, 2 Fat

SAVORY PITA CHIPS

MAKES 4 SERVINGS

1. Preheat oven to 350°F. Line baking sheet with foil.

2. Carefully cut each pita round in half horizontally; split into two rounds. Cut each round into six wedges.

3. Place wedges, inside layer down, on prepared baking sheet. Spray with cooking spray. Turn over; spray again.

4. Combine Parmesan cheese, basil and garlic powder in small bowl; sprinkle evenly over pita wedges.

5. Bake 12 to 14 minutes or until golden brown. Cool completely.

CINNAMON CRISPS: Substitute butter-flavored cooking spray for olive oil cooking spray and 1 tablespoon sugar mixed with ¼ teaspoon ground cinnamon for Parmesan cheese, basil and garlic powder.

2 whole wheat or white pita bread rounds

Olive oil cooking spray

3 tablespoons grated Parmesan cheese

1 teaspoon dried basil

¼ teaspoon garlic powder

Calories 108, **Total Fat** 2g, **Saturated Fat** 1g, **Cholesterol** 4mg, **Sodium** 257mg, Carbohydrates 18g, **Dietary Fiber** 2g, **Protein** 5g
Dietary Exchanges: 1 Bread/Starch, ½ Meat

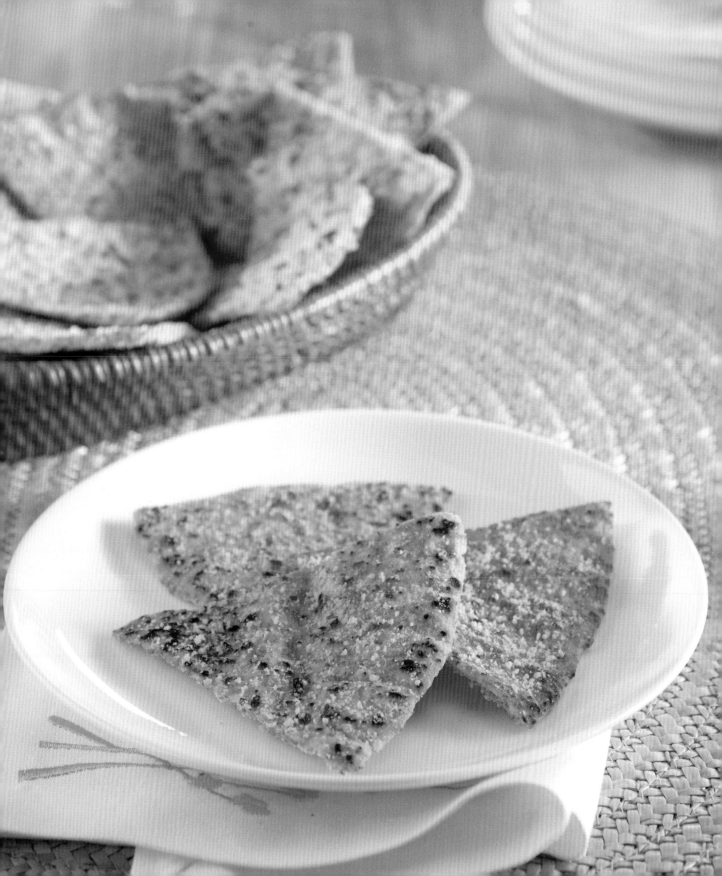

KIWI & STRAWBERRIES WITH PINE NUTS

MAKES 4 SERVINGS

1. Peel kiwi; slice each into 6 thin rounds. Arrange 3 slices kiwi on four dessert plates.

2. Wash, hull and slice strawberries. Arrange strawberries evenly over kiwi slices. Drizzle orange juice evenly over each dish. Top evenly with pine nuts.

2 kiwi fruits

1½ cups fresh strawberries

1 tablespoon orange juice

1 tablespoon pine nuts,* toasted

To toast pine nuts, cook and stir in small skillet over medium heat 3 minutes or until lightly browned.

Calories 90, **Total Fat** 5g, **Saturated Fat** 1g, **Cholesterol** 0mg, **Sodium** 0mg, **Carbohydrates** 11g, **Dietary Fiber** 3g, **Protein** 2g
Dietary Exchanges: ½ Fruit, 1 Fat

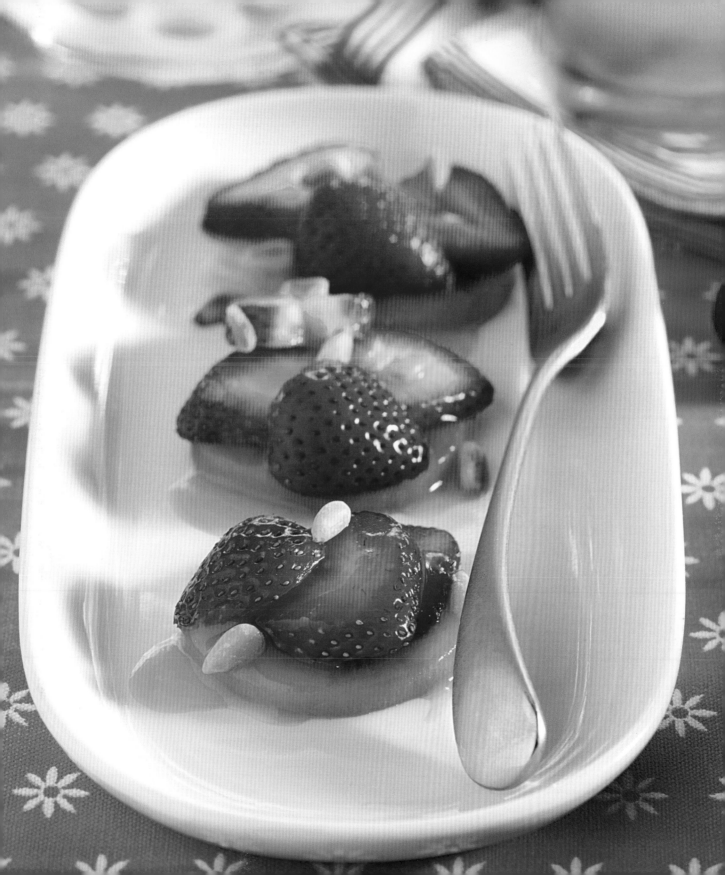

CHERRY TOMATO POPS

MAKES 8 POPS

1. Slice cheese sticks in half lengthwise. Trim stem end of each cherry tomato and remove pulp and seeds.

2. Press end of cheese stick into hollowed tomato to make cherry tomato pop. Serve with ranch dressing for dipping.

4 part-skim mozzarella string cheese sticks (1 ounce each)

8 cherry tomatoes

3 tablespoons fat-free ranch dressing

Calories 56, **Total Fat** 3g, **Saturated Fat** 2g, **Cholesterol** 10mg, **Sodium** 210mg, **Carbohydrates** 4g, **Dietary Fiber** 1g, **Protein** 3g
Dietary Exchanges: 1/2 Meat, 1/2 Vegetable

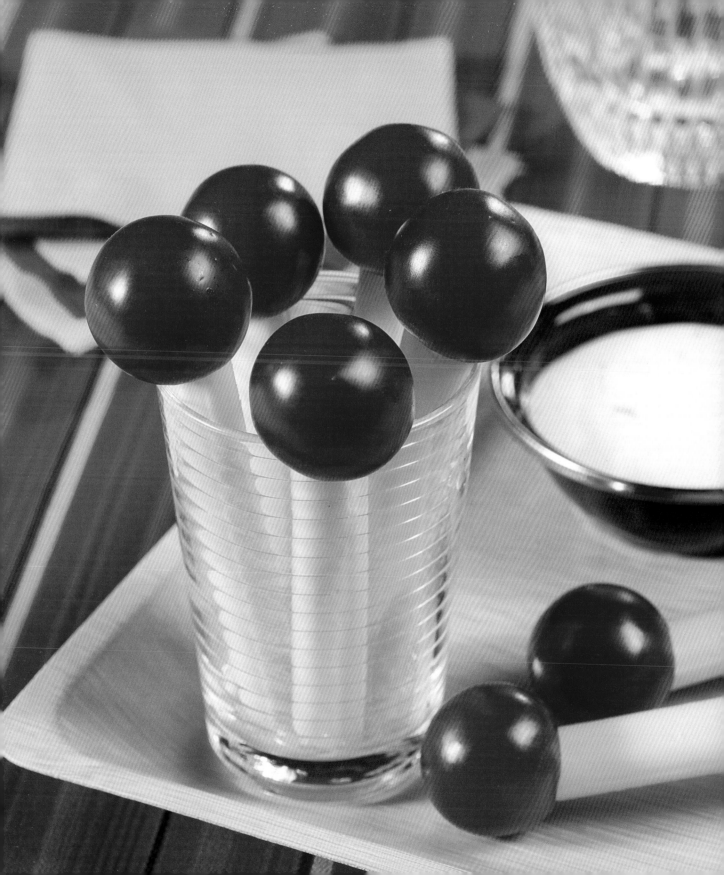

BITE-YOU-BACK ROASTED EDAMAME

MAKES 4 ($1/2$-CUP) SERVINGS

1. Preheat oven to 375°F.

2. Combine oil, honey and wasabi powder in large bowl; mix well. Add edamame; toss to coat. Spread on baking sheet in single layer.

3. Bake 12 to 15 minutes or until golden brown, stirring once. Immediately remove from baking sheet to large bowl; sprinkle generously with salt, if desired. Cool completely before serving. Store in airtight container.

2 **teaspoons vegetable oil**

2 **teaspoons honey**

$1/4$ **teaspoon wasabi powder***

1 **package (10 ounces) shelled edamame, thawed if frozen**

Kosher salt (optional)

*This ingredient can be found in the Asian section of most supermarkets and in Asian specialty markets.

Calories 120, **Total Fat** 6g, **Saturated Fat** 0g, **Cholesterol** 0mg, **Sodium** 5mg, **Carbohydrates** 9g, **Dietary Fiber** 4g, **Protein** 10g
Dietary Exchanges: $1/2$ Bread/Starch, 1 Meat, $1/2$ Fat

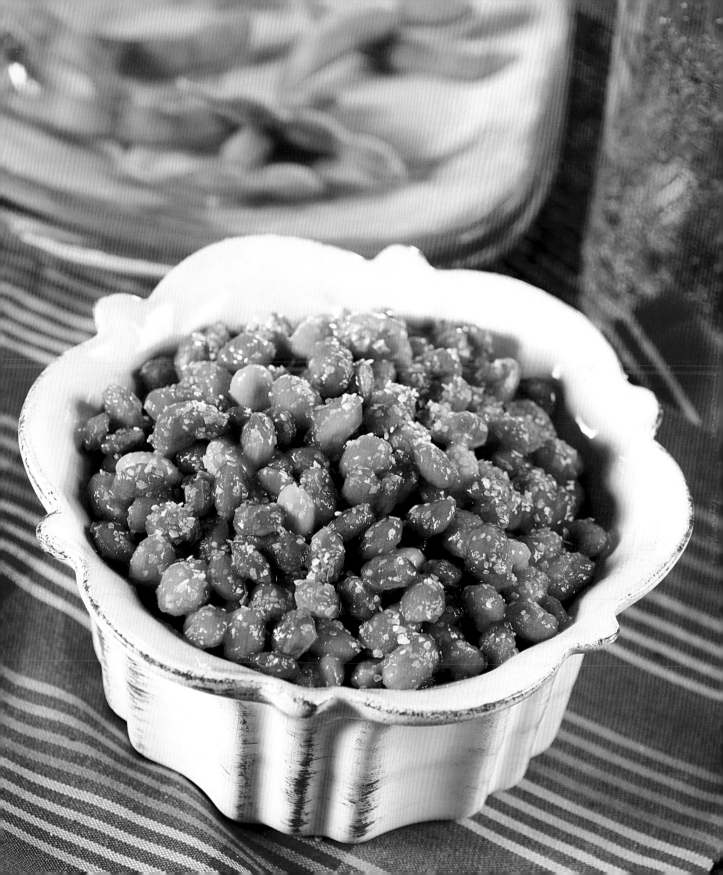

PEPPY SNACK MIX

MAKES 6 ($^2/_3$-CUP) SERVINGS

Preheat oven to 300°F. Combine rice cake pieces, cereal and pretzels in 13×9-inch baking pan. Combine margarine, Worcestershire sauce, chili powder and red pepper in small bowl. Drizzle over cereal mixture; toss to combine. Bake 20 minutes, stirring after 10 minutes.

- 3 (3-inch) plain rice cakes, broken into bite-size pieces
- 1$^1/_2$ cups bite-size frosted shredded wheat cereal
- $^3/_4$ cup pretzel sticks, halved
- 3 tablespoons reduced-fat margarine, melted
- 2 teaspoons reduced-sodium Worcestershire sauce
- $^3/_4$ teaspoon chili powder
- $^1/_8$ to $^1/_4$ teaspoon ground red pepper

Calories 118, **Total Fat** 3g, **Saturated Fat** 1g, **Cholesterol** 0mg, **Sodium** 156mg, **Carbohydrates** 20g, **Dietary Fiber** 1g, **Protein** 2g
Dietary Exchanges: 1$^1/_2$ Bread/Starch, $^1/_2$ Fat

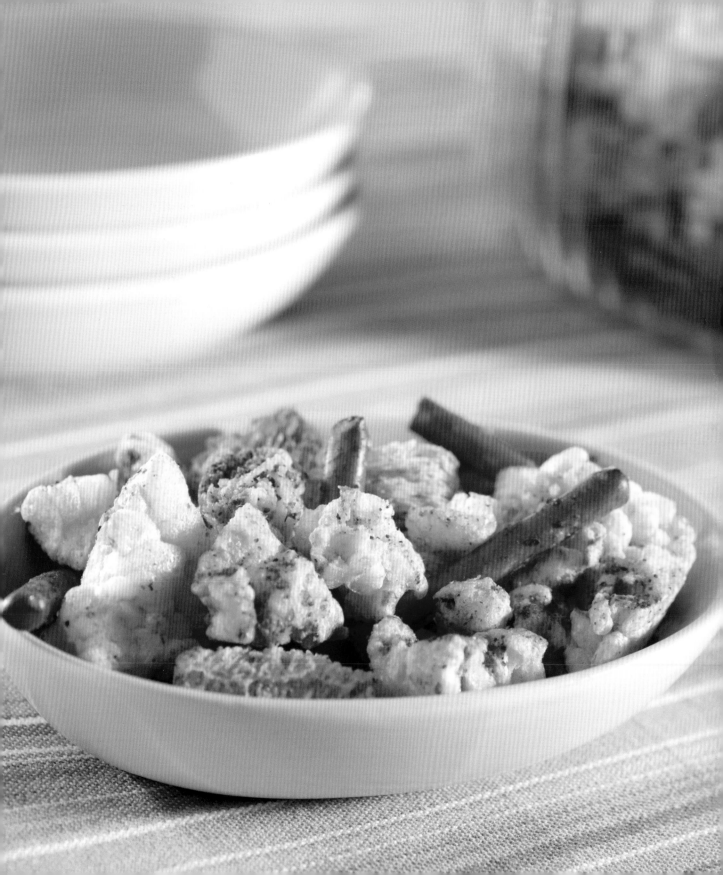

DOUBLE MELON POPS

MAKES 5 SERVINGS

1. Combine honeydew and 2 teaspoons lime juice in blender or food processor; blend until smooth.

2. Spoon about ¼ cup honeydew mixture evenly into ice pop molds or 5-ounce paper cups and freeze 1 hour.

3. Combine cantaloupe and remaining 2 teaspoons lime juice in blender or food processor; blend until smooth. Top honeydew layer evenly with cantaloupe mixture. Insert handles of ice pop molds or insert pop stick into cups. Freeze 4 hours or until firm.

2 cups honeydew chunks (1-inch)

4 teaspoons lime juice, divided

2 cups cantaloupe chunks (1-inch)

Calories 48, **Total Fat** 0g, **Saturated Fat** 0g, **Cholesterol** 0mg, **Sodium** 23mg, **Carbohydrates** 12g, **Dietary Fiber** 1g, **Protein** 1g
Dietary Exchanges: 1 Fruit

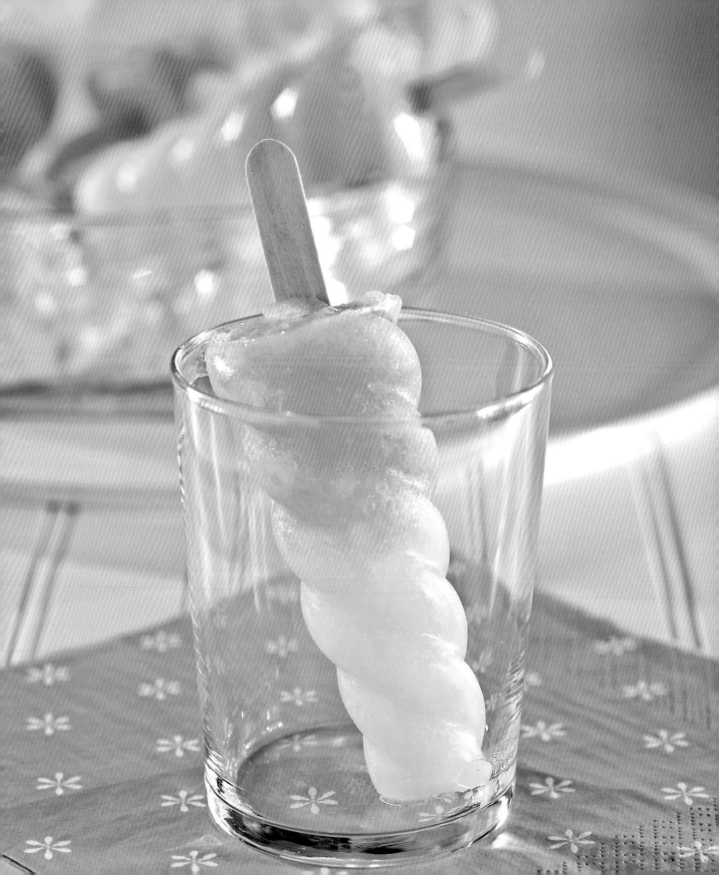

SNACK ATTACK MIX

MAKES 16 (1/2-CUP) SERVINGS

1. Preheat oven to 300°F. Combine cereal, pretzels, pita chips and almonds in large bowl; set aside.

2. Combine remaining ingredients in small bowl; stir until well blended. Spoon over cereal mixture; toss gently, yet thoroughly, to coat completely. Spread evenly on large baking sheet. Bake 10 to 15 minutes or until beginning to lightly brown, stirring every 5 minutes.

3. Remove from oven; place baking sheet on wire rack. Let stand 2 hours. Store leftovers in an airtight container at room temperature.

- 4 cups unsweetened corn cereal squares or whole wheat cereal squares
- 1 1/2 ounces (3/4 cup) fat-free pretzels sticks, broken in half
- 1 1/2 ounces (1 cup) multigrain pita chips, broken into bite-size pieces
- 4 ounces (about 1 cup) slivered almonds
- 2 teaspoons paprika
- 1 teaspoon dry mustard
- 1 teaspoon garlic powder
- 1 teaspoon salt
- 1/2 teaspoon ground cumin
- 1/4 teaspoon ground red pepper
- 2 tablespoons Worcestershire sauce
- 2 teaspoons canola oil
- 1 1/2 teaspoons cider vinegar

Calories 99, **Total Fat** 5g, **Saturated Fat** 0g, **Cholesterol** 0mg, **Sodium** 279mg, **Carbohydrates** 12g, **Dietary Fiber** 2g, **Protein** 3g
Dietary Exchanges: 1 Bread/Starch, 1 Fat

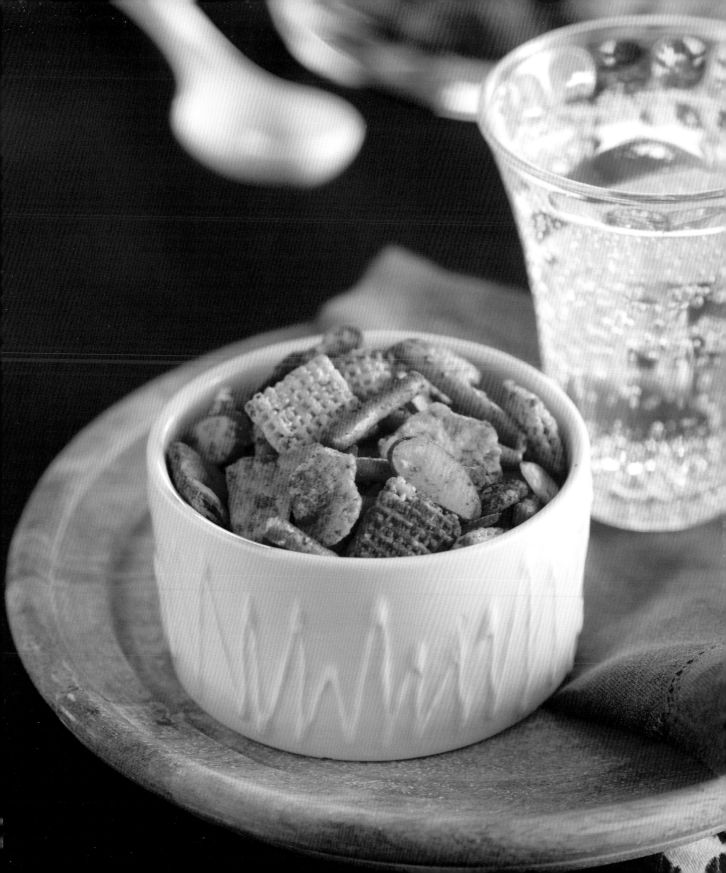

GREAT ZUKES PIZZA BITES

MAKES 8 SERVINGS

1. Preheat broiler; set rack 4 inches from heat.

2. Trim and discard ends of zucchini. Cut zucchini into 16 (¼-inch-thick) diagonal slices. Place on nonstick baking sheet.

3. Combine pizza sauce, tomato paste and oregano in small bowl; mix well. Spread scant teaspoon sauce over each zucchini slice. Combine cheeses in small bowl. Top each zucchini slice with 1 tablespoon cheese mixture, pressing down into sauce. Place 1 olive slice on each of 8 pizza bites. Place 1 folded pepperoni slice on each remaining pizza bite.

4. Broil 3 minutes or until cheese is melted. Serve immediately.

1 medium zucchini

3 tablespoons pizza sauce

2 tablespoons tomato paste

¼ teaspoon dried oregano

¾ cup (3 ounces) shredded mozzarella cheese

¼ cup shredded Parmesan cheese

8 slices pitted black olives

8 slices pepperoni

Calories 75, **Total Fat** 5g, **Saturated Fat** 2g, **Cholesterol** 10mg, **Sodium** 288mg, **Carbohydrates** 3g, **Dietary Fiber** 1g, **Protein** 5g
Dietary Exchanges: ½ Meat, ½ Vegetable, 1 Fat

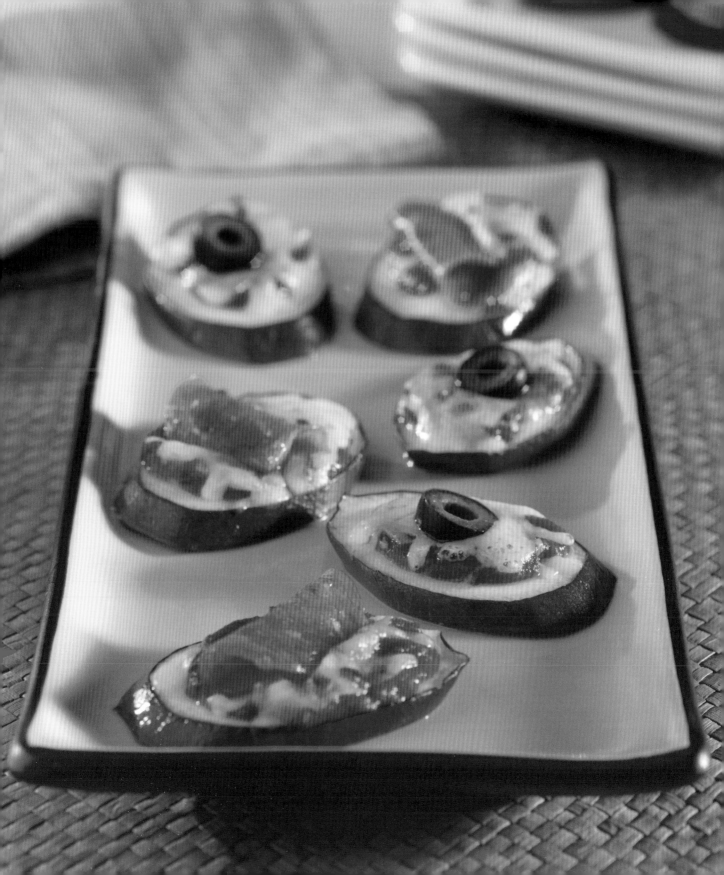

POPCORN GRANOLA

MAKES 8 SERVINGS

1. Preheat oven to 350°F. Spread oats on ungreased baking sheet; bake 10 to 15 minutes or until lightly toasted, stirring occasionally.

2. Combine oats, popcorn, raisins, dried fruit and sunflower kernels in large bowl. Heat butter, brown sugar, honey, cinnamon and nutmeg in small saucepan over medium heat until butter is melted. Drizzle over popcorn mixture; toss to coat.

1 cup quick oats

6 cups air-popped popcorn

1 cup golden raisins

$\frac{1}{2}$ cup chopped mixed dried fruit

$\frac{1}{4}$ cup sunflower kernels

2 tablespoons butter

2 tablespoons packed light brown sugar

1 tablespoon honey

$\frac{1}{4}$ teaspoon ground cinnamon

$\frac{1}{4}$ teaspoon ground nutmeg

Calories 218, **Total Fat** 6g, **Saturated Fat** 1g, **Cholesterol** 0mg, **Sodium** 38mg, **Carbohydrates** 40g, **Dietary Fiber** 3g, **Protein** 5g
Dietary Exchanges: $\frac{1}{2}$ Bread/Starch, 2 Fruit, 1 Fat

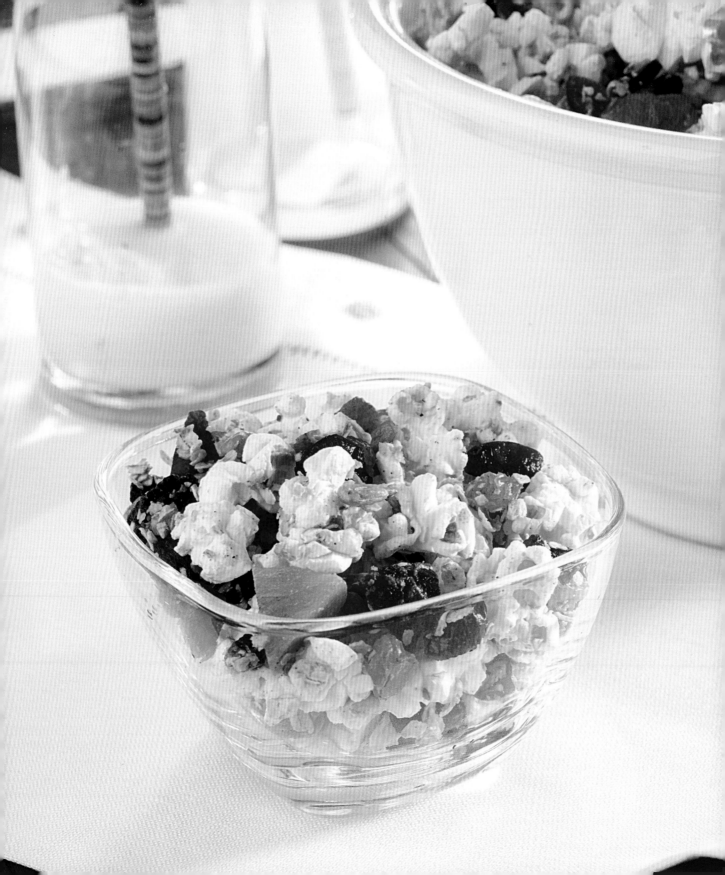

BEET CHIPS

MAKES 3 SERVINGS

1. Preheat oven to 300°F.

2. Cut beets into very thin slices, about $^1/_{16}$ inch thick. Combine beets, oil, salt and pepper in medium bowl; gently toss to coat. Arrange in single layer on baking sheets.

3. Bake 30 to 35 minutes or until darkened and crisp.* Spread on paper towels to cool completely.

*If the beet chips are darkened but not crisp, turn oven off and let chips stand in oven until crisp, about 10 minutes. Do not keep the oven on as the chips will burn easily.

3 medium beets (red and/or golden), trimmed

$1^1/_2$ tablespoons extra virgin olive oil

$^1/_4$ teaspoon salt

$^1/_4$ teaspoon black pepper

Calories 100, **Total Fat** 7g, **Saturated Fat** 1g, **Cholesterol** 0mg, **Sodium** 260mg, **Carbohydrates** 8g, **Dietary Fiber** 2g, **Protein** 1g
Dietary Exchanges: 2 Vegetable, 2 Fat

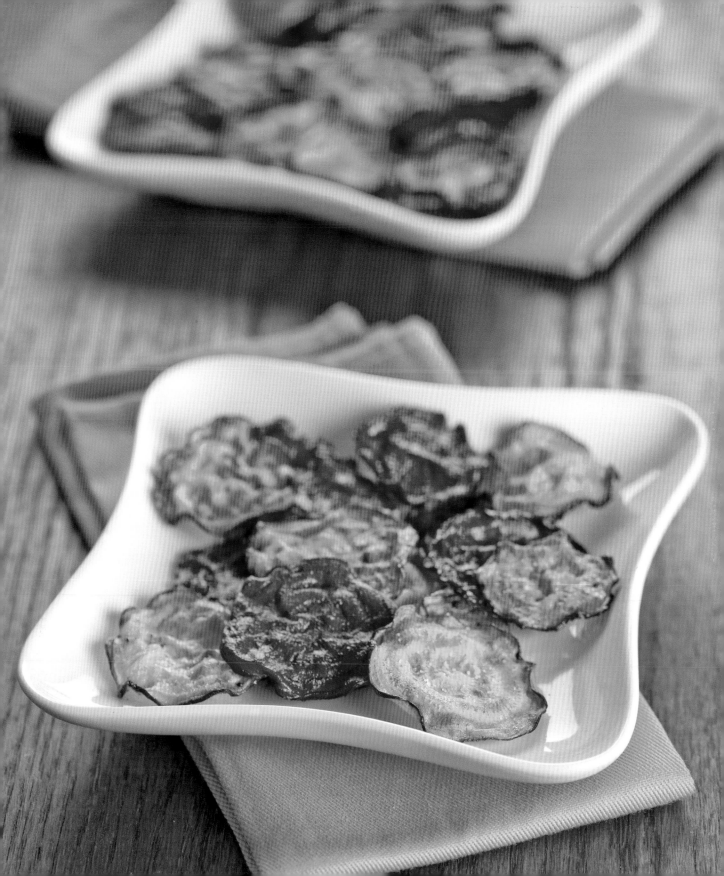

PEANUT PITAS

MAKES 8 SERVINGS

1. Spread inside of each pita half with 1 teaspoon peanut butter and 1 teaspoon fruit spread.

2. Fill pita halves evenly with banana slices. Serve immediately.

HONEY BEES: Substitute honey for fruit spread.

JOLLY JELLIES: Substitute any flavor jelly for fruit spread and thin apple slices for banana slices.

P. B. CRUNCHERS: Substitute reduced-fat mayonnaise for fruit spread and celery slices for banana slices.

1 package (8 ounces) small pita bread rounds, cut into halves

16 teaspoons reduced-fat peanut butter

16 teaspoons strawberry fruit spread

1 large banana, peeled and thinly sliced (about 48 slices)

Calories 167, **Total Fat** 5g, **Saturated Fat** 1g, **Cholesterol** 0mg, **Sodium** 177mg, **Carbohydrates** 26g, **Dietary Fiber** 1g, **Protein** 6g
Dietary Exchanges: 2 Bread/Starch, 1/2 Fat

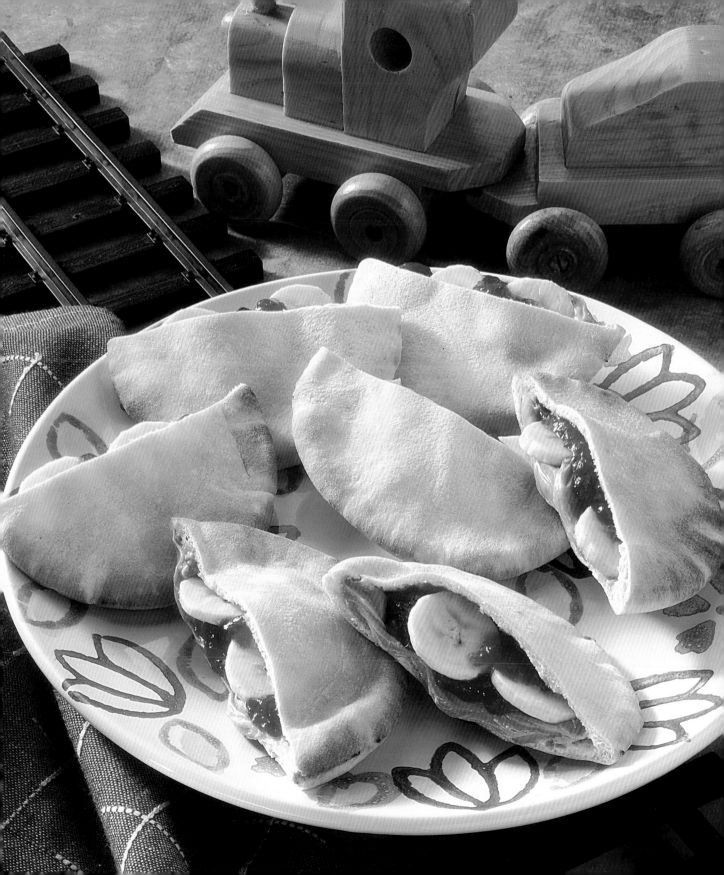

TORTELLINI TEASERS

MAKES 6 SERVINGS

1. Prepare Zesty Tomato Sauce; keep warm.

2. Cook tortellini according to package directions. Drain.

3. Alternately thread tortellini and vegetable pieces on wooden skewers. Serve as dippers with Zesty Tomato Sauce.

Zesty Tomato Sauce (recipe follows)

$1/2$ (9-ounce) package refrigerated cheese tortellini

1 large red or green bell pepper, cut into 1-inch pieces

2 medium carrots, cut into $1/2$-inch pieces

1 medium zucchini, cut into $1/2$-inch pieces

12 medium mushrooms

12 cherry tomatoes

ZESTY TOMATO SAUCE

MAKES ABOUT $1^2/_3$ CUPS

Combine tomato purée, onion, parsley, oregano and thyme in small saucepan. Heat thoroughly, stirring occasionally. Stir in salt and black pepper.

1 can (15 ounces) tomato purée

2 tablespoons finely chopped onion

2 tablespoons chopped fresh parsley

1 teaspoon dried oregano

$1/_4$ teaspoon dried thyme

$1/_4$ teaspoon salt

$1/_8$ teaspoon black pepper

Calories 130, **Total Fat** 2g, **Saturated Fat** 1g, **Cholesterol** 12mg, **Sodium** 306mg, **Carbohydrates** 23g, **Dietary Fiber** 5g, **Protein** 7g
Dietary Exchanges: 1 Bread/Starch, 2 Vegetable

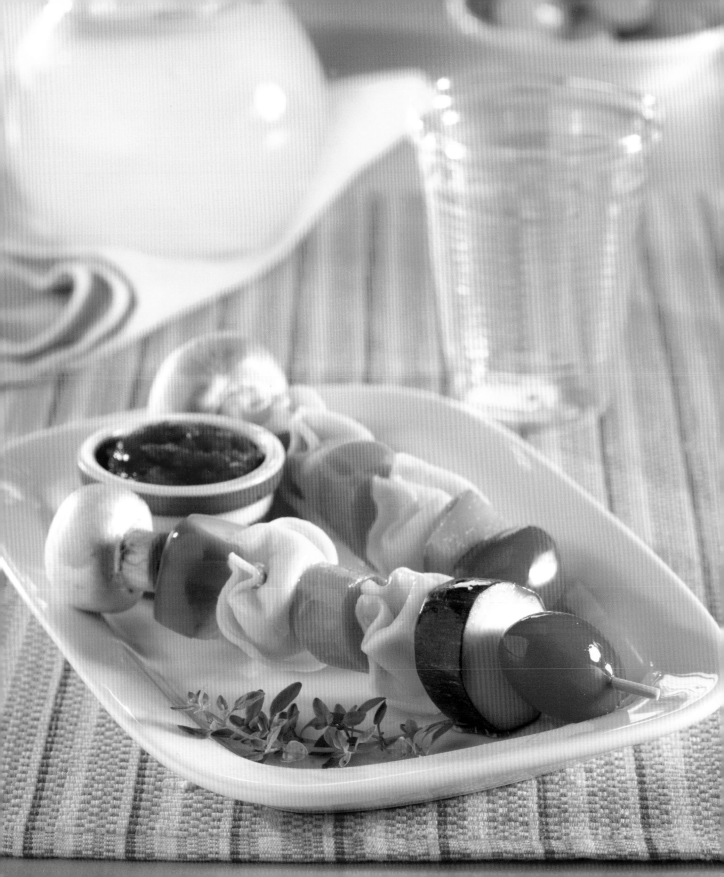

BANANA FREEZER POPS

MAKES 8 SERVINGS

1. Combine bananas, orange juice concentrate, water, honey and vanilla in blender or food processor; blend until smooth.

2. Pour banana mixture evenly into cups; cover top of each cup with a small piece of foil. Insert pop stick into banana mixture through center of foil.

3. Place cups on tray; freeze about 3 hours or until firm. To serve, remove foil and paper cups.

PEPPY PURPLE POPS: Omit honey and vanilla. Substitute grape juice concentrate for orange juice concentrate.

FROZEN BANANA SHAKES: Increase water to $1\frac{1}{2}$ cups. Prepare fruit mixture as directed. Add 4 ice cubes; process on high speed until mixture is thick and creamy. Makes 3 servings.

2 ripe medium bananas, cut into chunks

1 can (6 ounces) frozen orange juice concentrate

$\frac{1}{4}$ cup water

1 tablespoon honey

1 teaspoon vanilla

8 (3-ounce) paper or plastic cups

8 pop sticks

Calories 83, **Total Fat** 1g, **Saturated Fat** 1g, **Cholesterol** 0mg, **Sodium** 1mg, **Carbohydrates** 20g, **Dietary Fiber** 1g, **Protein** 1g
Dietary Exchanges: $1\frac{1}{2}$ Fruit

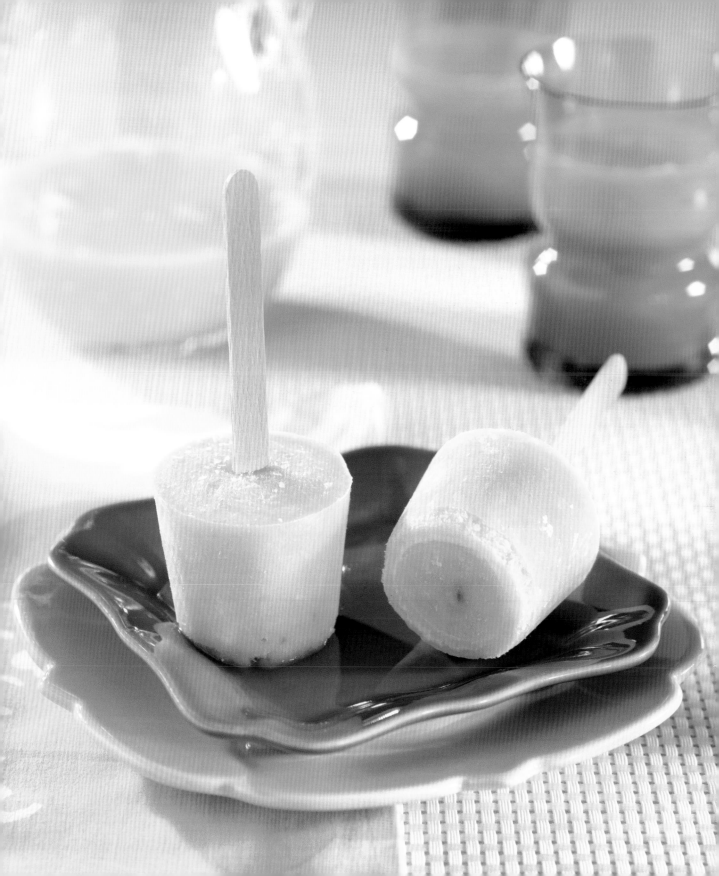

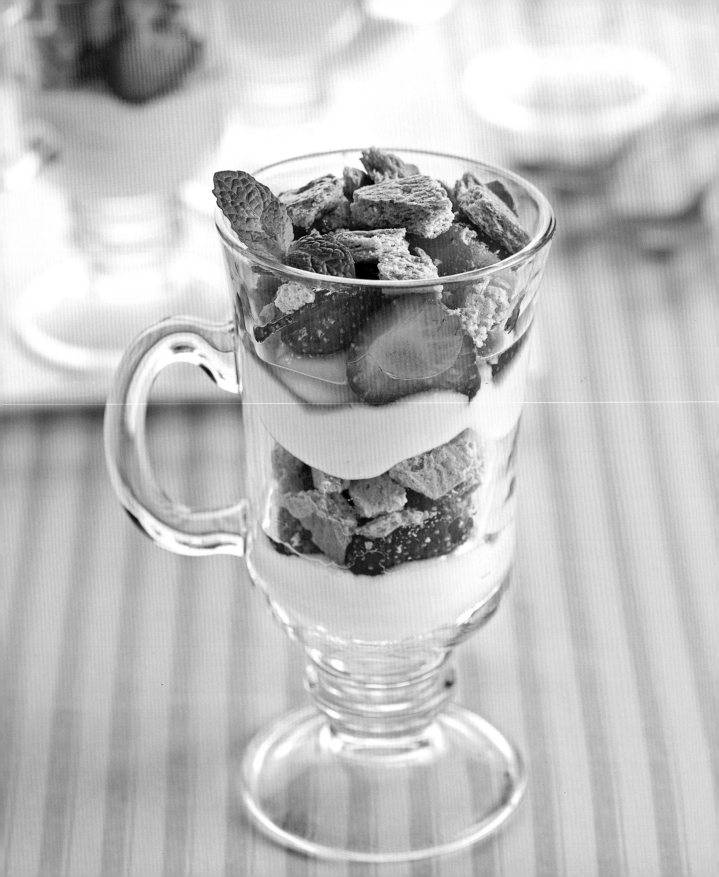

DELICIOUS DESSERTS

STRAWBERRY CHEESECAKE PARFAITS

MAKES 4 SERVINGS

1. Whisk yogurt, cream cheese, powdered sugar and vanilla in small bowl until smooth and well blended.

2. Combine strawberries and granulated sugar in small bowl; gently toss.

3. Layer 1/4 cup yogurt mixture, 1/4 cup strawberries and 1/4 cup graham cracker crumbs in each of four dessert dishes. Repeat layers. Garnish with mint. Serve immediately.

1 1/2 cups vanilla nonfat Greek yogurt

1/2 cup whipped cream cheese, at room temperature

2 tablespoons powdered sugar

1 teaspoon vanilla

2 cups sliced fresh strawberries

2 teaspoons granulated sugar

8 honey graham cracker squares, coarsely crumbled (about 2 cups)

Fresh mint leaves (optional)

Calories 220, **Total Fat** 7g, **Saturated Fat** 3g, **Cholesterol** 15mg, **Sodium** 200mg, **Carbohydrates** 29g, **Dietary Fiber** 2g, **Protein** 11g
Dietary Exchanges: 1 Bread/Starch, 1 Meat, 1 Fruit, 1 Fat

FROZEN PINEAPPLE FUDGE

MAKES 4 (1/4-CUP) SERVINGS

Combine milk powder, cocoa and sugar substitute in medium bowl. Stir in pineapple until well combined. Pour into custard cups or ice cube trays; freeze 3 hours or until firm.

- 2/3 cup nonfat dry milk powder
- 4 teaspoons unsweetened cocoa powder
- 4 teaspoons sugar substitute*
- 1 cup unsweetened crushed canned pineapple

This recipe was tested using sucralose-based sugar substitute.

Calories 83, **Total Fat** 1g, **Saturated Fat** 1g, **Cholesterol** 2mg, **Sodium** 65mg, **Carbohydrates** 17g, **Dietary Fiber** 1g, **Protein** 5g
Dietary Exchanges: 1 Bread/Starch

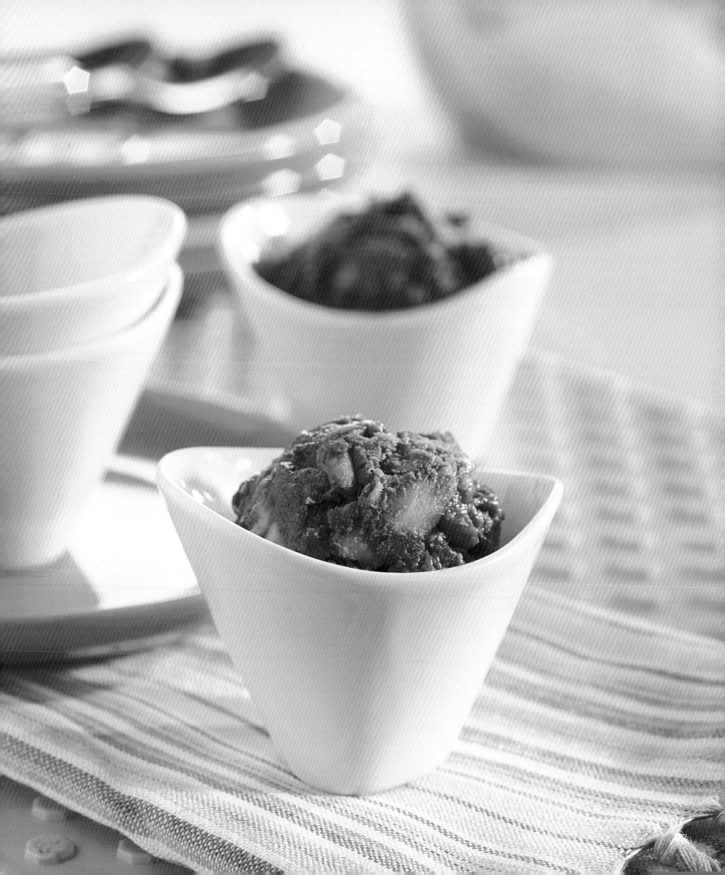

CHOCOLATE CREAM DESSERT DIP

MAKES 24 SERVINGS

1. Beat milk and pudding mix in medium bowl with electric mixer at medium speed 2 minutes.

2. Stir in whipped topping and chocolate chips until well blended. Refrigerate until ready to serve. Serve with fresh fruit or angel food cake for dipping.

2 cups fat-free (skim) milk

1 package (4-serving size) chocolate fat-free sugar-free instant pudding and pie filling mix

1 container (8 ounces) thawed fat-free whipped topping

2 tablespoons chocolate chips, finely chopped

Calories 33, **Total Fat** 1g, **Saturated Fat** 1g, **Cholesterol** 1mg, **Sodium** 38mg, **Carbohydrates** 6g, **Dietary Fiber** 0g, **Protein** 1g
Dietary Exchanges: 1/2 Bread/Starch
(*nutrition information for dip only*)

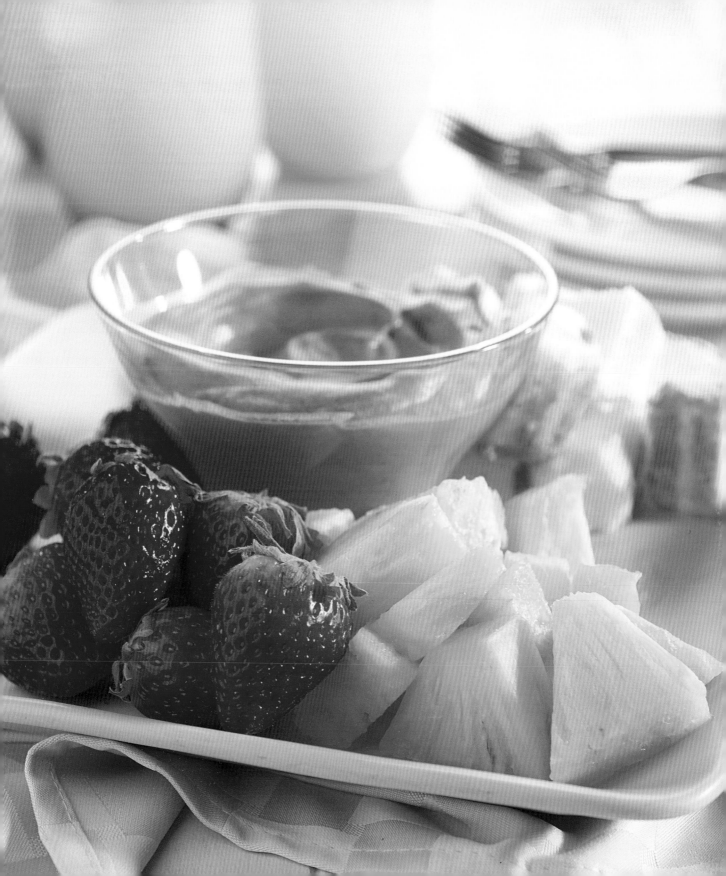

CRISPY NO-BAKE PEANUT BUTTER OAT COOKIES

MAKES 24 COOKIES (2 COOKIES PER SERVING)

1. Whisk sugar substitute, brown sugar, peanut butter, milk and margarine in large saucepan. Bring to a boil over medium-high heat; boil 1 minute.

2. Remove from heat. Stir in vanilla and oats; let stand 1 minute. Stir in rice cereal.

3. Drop mixture by tablespoons onto baking sheet lined with parchment paper. Refrigerate 20 minutes or until firm.

$^1/_2$ cup sugar substitute*

$^1/_2$ cup dark brown sugar (not packed)

6 tablespoons peanut butter

$^1/_4$ cup low-fat (1%) milk

2 tablespoons margarine

$^3/_4$ teaspoon vanilla

1 cup old-fashioned oats

1 cup crisp rice cereal

This recipe was tested using sucralose-based sugar substitute.

Calories 134, **Total Fat** 6g, **Saturated Fat** 1g, **Cholesterol** 1mg, **Sodium** 81mg, **Carbohydrates** 18g, **Dietary Fiber** 1g, **Protein** 3g
Dietary Exchanges: 1 Bread/Starch, 1 Fat

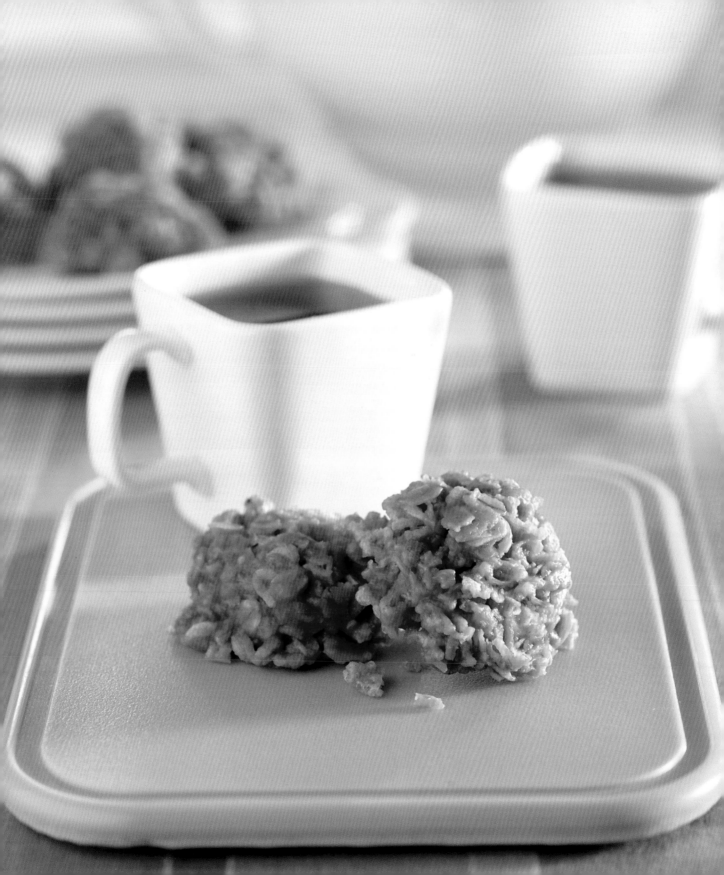

BANANAS FOSTER SUNDAE

MAKES 4 SERVINGS ($1/2$ CUP ICE CREAM
AND 2 TABLESPOONS TOPPING PER SERVING)

1. Peel banana; cut into 1/4-inch slices.

2. Heat brown sugar and butter in medium nonstick skillet over medium-low heat, stirring constantly. Stir in water; cook and stir 30 to 45 seconds or until slightly thickened. Add banana and rum extract, stirring gently to coat in caramel mixture. Cook about 30 seconds or until banana is heated through. Remove from heat.

3. Scoop ice cream into four individual dessert dishes; spoon banana mixture evenly over ice cream. Garnish with wafer cookie pieces, if desired. Serve immediately.

1 medium banana

2 tablespoons packed brown sugar

2 teaspoons butter

1 tablespoon water

1 teaspoon rum extract

2 cups vanilla sugar-free reduced-fat ice cream

Wafer cookie pieces (optional)

Calories 180, **Total Fat** 7g, **Saturated Fat** 4g, **Cholesterol** 25mg, **Sodium** 70mg, **Carbohydrates** 28g, **Dietary Fiber** 1g, **Protein** 3g
Dietary Exchanges: 1 1/2 Bread/Starch, 1/2 Fruit, 1 1/2 Fat

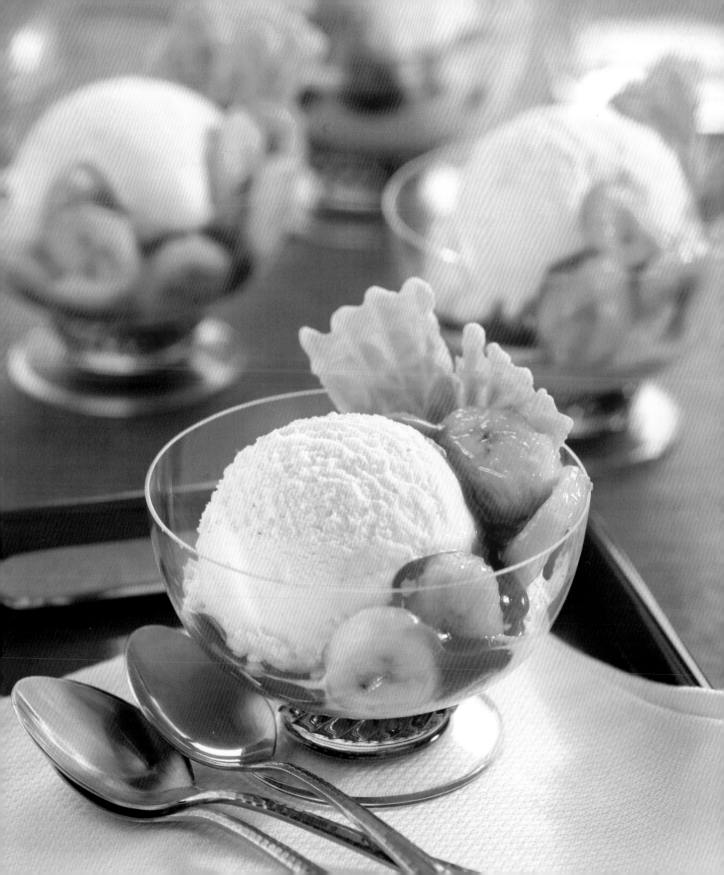

CHOCOLATE-DRIZZLED FROZEN GRAPES

MAKES 2 SERVINGS

1. Wash grapes; remove from stems. Dry completely with paper towel. Place in single layer on baking sheet. Freeze 2 hours or up to 48 hours.

2. About 5 minutes before serving, place chocolate chips and milk in small microwavable cup. Microwave on HIGH 20 seconds; stir until chocolate is melted. Microwave in 10-second intervals, if necessary, until chocolate is melted and smooth.

3. Remove grapes from freezer. Divide evenly into two small dessert dishes. Sprinkle with powdered sugar. Drizzle melted chocolate over grapes. Garnish with mint. Serve immediately.

NOTE: To drizzle chocolate, place melted chocolate mixture in resealable food storage bag. Snip corner of bag and squeeze chocolate over grapes.

1 cup seedless grapes (green and red)

1 tablespoon semisweet chocolate chips

1 teaspoon fat-free (skim) milk

$\frac{1}{2}$ teaspoon powdered sugar

Fresh mint (optional)

Calories 81, **Total Fat** 2g, **Saturated Fat** 1g, **Cholesterol** 0mg, **Sodium** 3mg, **Carbohydrates** 18g, **Dietary Fiber** 1g, **Protein** 1g
Dietary Exchanges: 1 Fruit, $\frac{1}{2}$ Fat

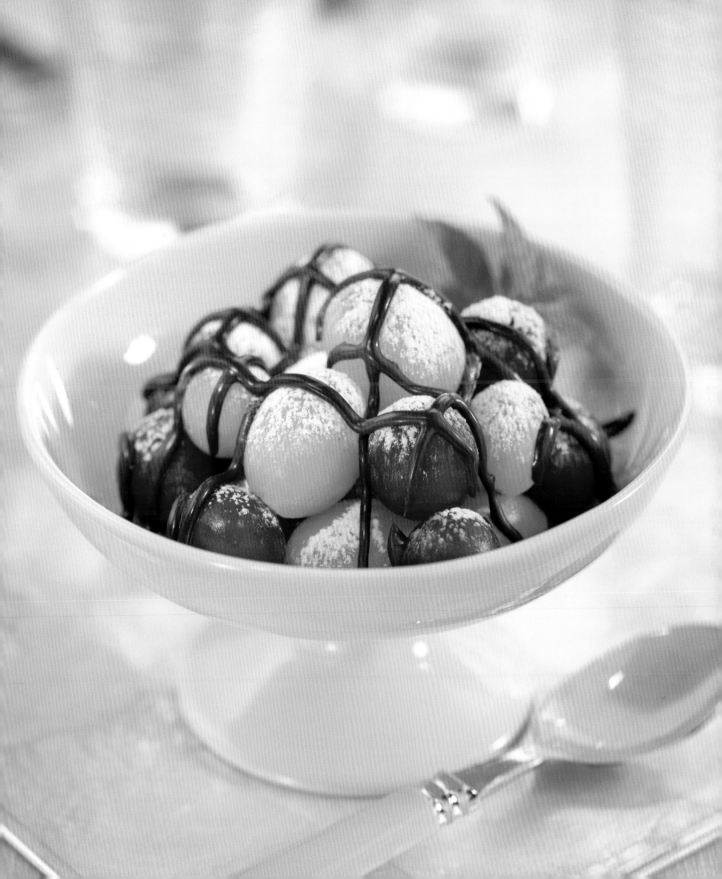

YOGURT "CUSTARD" WITH BLUEBERRIES

MAKES 1 SERVING

1. Spoon yogurt into paper towel-lined strainer. Place over bowl; refrigerate 20 minutes to drain and thicken.

2. Combine yogurt, honey and nutmeg in small bowl. Combine blueberries and preserves; spoon over yogurt. Top with almonds.

1 container (6 ounces) plain fat-free yogurt

2 teaspoons honey

1/8 teaspoon ground nutmeg

1/2 cup fresh or thawed frozen blueberries

1 tablespoon all fruit blueberry or raspberry preserves

1 tablespoon sliced almonds, toasted

Calories 261, **Total Fat** 3g, **Saturated Fat** 1g, **Cholesterol** 4mg, **Sodium** 137mg, **Carbohydrates** 49g, **Dietary Fiber** 3g, **Protein** 11g
Dietary Exchanges: 2 Fruit, 1 1/2 Milk

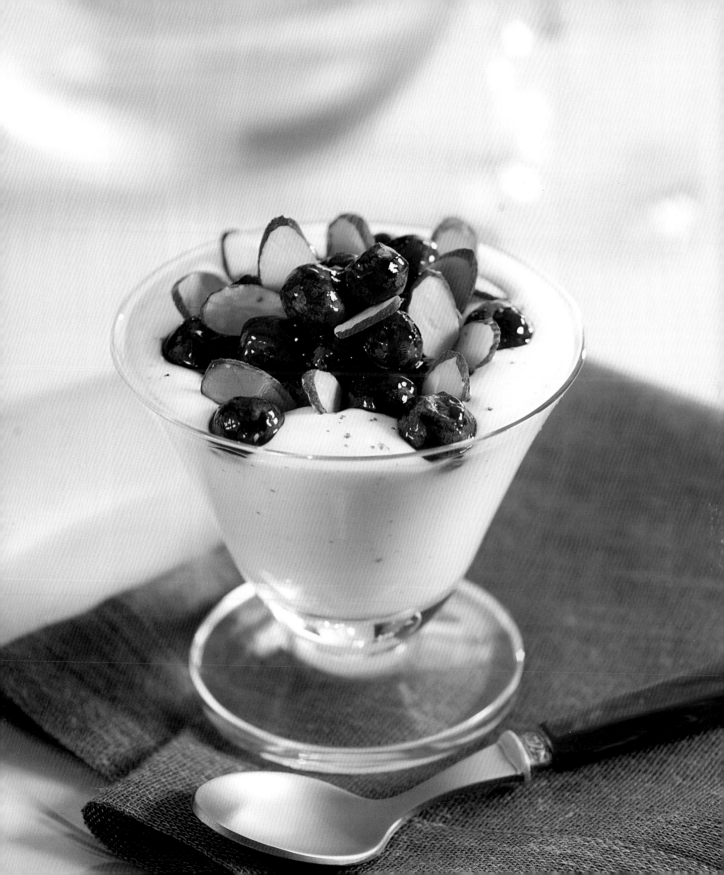

CHOCOLATE HAZELNUT MOUSSE

MAKES 8 SERVINGS

1. Prepare pudding with fat-free milk according to package directions. Whisk in hazelnut spread. Refrigerate 15 minutes.

2. Fold whipped topping into pudding. Spoon mixture into stemmed glasses or small ramekins or bowls. Refrigerate until ready to serve. Garnish with dollop of whipped topping and strawberries, if desired.

1 package (4-serving size) chocolate fat-free sugar-free instant pudding and pie filling mix

2 cups fat-free (skim) milk

1/2 cup chocolate hazelnut spread

1 1/2 cups light whipped topping, plus additional for garnish (optional)

Fresh strawberries, halved (optional)

Calories 166, **Total Fat** 7g, **Saturated Fat** 2g, **Cholesterol** 1mg, **Sodium** 176mg, **Carbohydrates** 21g, **Dietary Fiber** 1g, **Protein** 3g
Dietary Exchanges: 1 1/2 Bread/Starch, 1 1/2 Fat

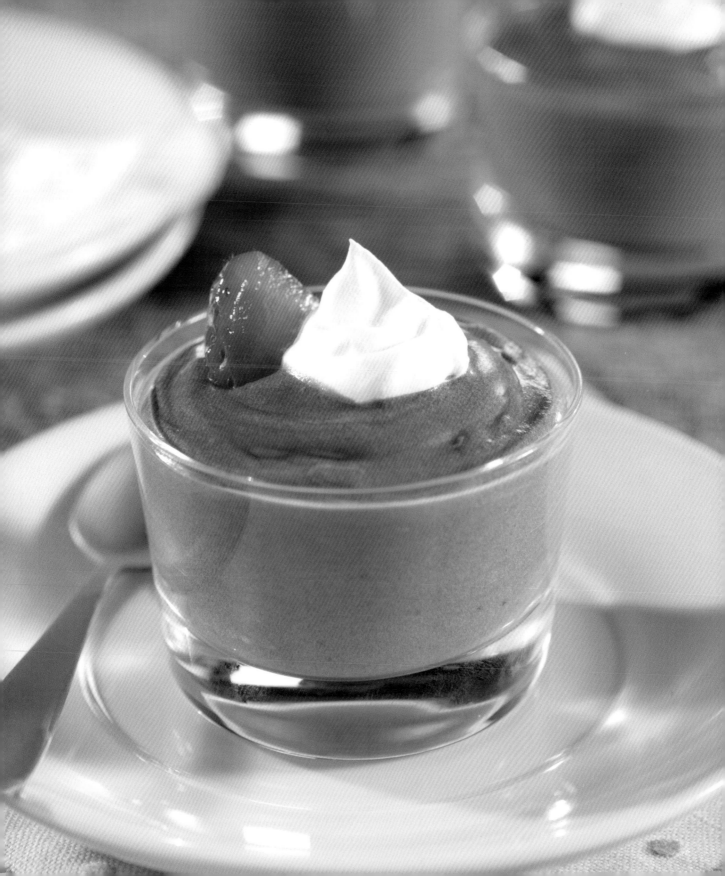

RASPBERRY AND CREAM FROZEN YOGURT PIE

MAKES 10 SERVINGS

1. Coat 9-inch pie plate with nonstick cooking spray; set aside.

2. Place graham crackers in resealable food storage bag; crush into fine crumbs with rolling pin. Mix crumbs and ¼ cup sugar substitute in small bowl. Stir in butter until crumbs are moistened. Press crumb crust into bottom and slightly up side of prepared pie plate. Refrigerate while making filling.

3. Beat cream cheese, yogurt, ⅓ cup sugar substitute and vanilla in bowl of electric mixer until combined. Add whipped topping; mix until just combined.

4. Spoon filling into crust and spread to edges. Freeze at least 4 hours or until frozen. Remove from freezer about 20 to 30 minutes before cutting into slices. Garnish with raspberries, if desired.

CRUST

7 chocolate graham crackers*

¼ cup sugar substitute**

3 to 4 tablespoons unsalted butter, melted

FILLING

1 package (8 ounces) fat-free cream cheese

1 container (6 ounces) raspberry low-fat yogurt

⅓ cup sugar substitute**

1 teaspoon vanilla

1 container (12 ounces) nonfat whipped topping, thawed

1 cup fresh raspberries (optional)

*If unavailable, may substitute with honey graham crackers.

**This recipe was tested using sucralose-based sugar substitute.

Calories 160, **Total Fat** 5g, **Saturated Fat** 3g, **Cholesterol** 12mg, **Sodium** 249mg, **Carbohydrates** 24g, **Dietary Fiber** 1g, **Protein** 5g
Dietary Exchanges: 1 Bread/Starch, ½ Fruit, 1 Fat

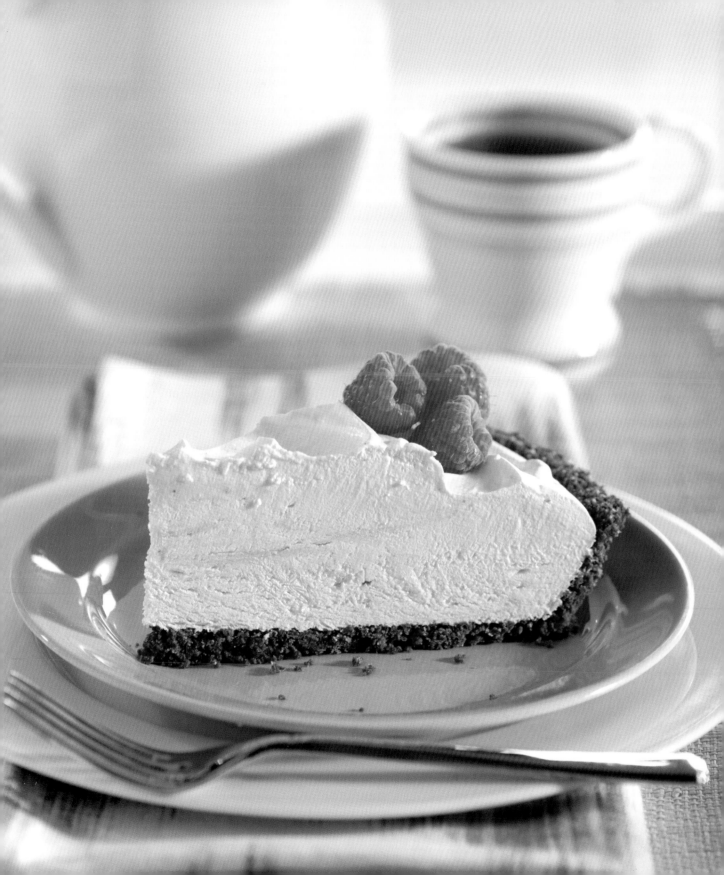

MARINATED PINEAPPLE DESSERT

MAKES 4 SERVINGS

1. Combine pineapple with juice, honey, cinnamon, lemon juice, vanilla and lemon peel in small saucepan. Bring to a boil over medium-high heat. Pour mixture into medium bowl; cover and refrigerate at least 4 hours or up to 24 hours.

2. Drain pineapple mixture; reserve liquid. Remove and discard cinnamon pieces.

3. Divide pineapple and strawberries evenly among four dessert dishes. Pour reserved liquid evenly over fruit. Sprinkle with coconut before serving.

1 can (20 ounces) pineapple chunks in juice, undrained

2 tablespoons honey

1 stick cinnamon, broken into pieces

1 tablespoon lemon juice

1 teaspoon vanilla

1/2 teaspoon grated lemon peel

1 1/2 cups fresh strawberries, cut into halves

1/4 cup flaked coconut, toasted*

*To toast coconut, spread in single layer in heavy-bottomed skillet. Cook over medium heat 1 to 2 minutes until lightly browned, stirring frequently. Remove from skillet immediately. Cool before using.

Calories 167, **Total Fat** 3g, **Saturated Fat** 1g, **Cholesterol** 0mg, **Sodium** 14mg, **Carbohydrates** 38g, **Dietary Fiber** 2g, **Protein** 1g
Dietary Exchanges: 2 1/2 Fruit, 1/2 Fat

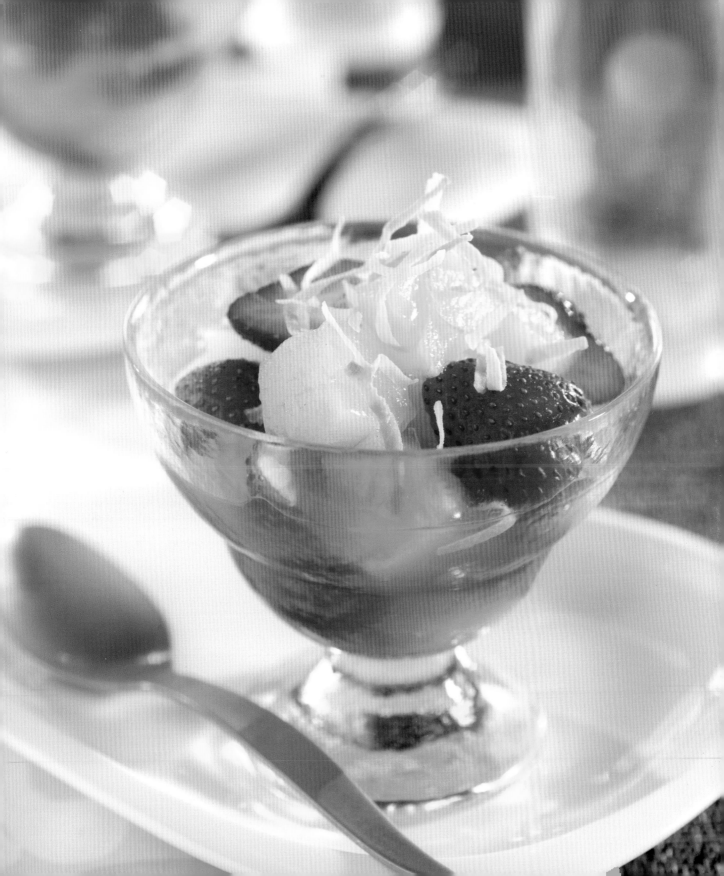

CINNAMON PEAR CRISP

MAKES 12 SERVINGS

1. Preheat oven to 375°F. Spray 11×7-inch baking dish with nonstick cooking spray.

2. Combine pears, apple juice concentrate, raisins, 3 tablespoons flour and cinnamon in large bowl; mix well. Transfer to prepared baking dish.

3. Combine oats, remaining ¼ cup flour, brown sugar and margarine in medium bowl; stir until mixture resembles coarse crumbs. Sprinkle evenly over pear mixture.

4. Bake 1 hour or until topping is golden brown.

- 8 pears, peeled and sliced
- ¾ cup unsweetened apple juice concentrate
- ½ cup golden raisins
- ¼ cup plus 3 tablespoons all-purpose flour, divided
- 1 teaspoon ground cinnamon
- ⅓ cup quick oats
- 3 tablespoons packed dark brown sugar
- 3 tablespoons margarine, melted

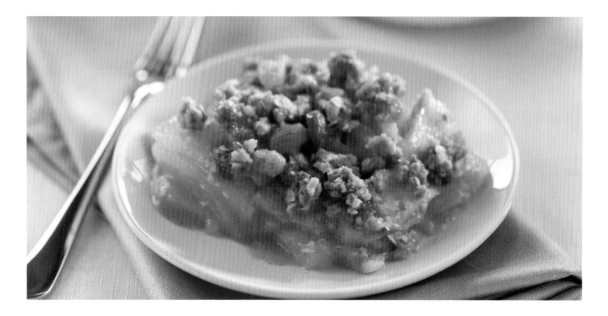

Calories 179, **Total Fat** 4g, **Saturated Fat** 1g, **Cholesterol** 0mg, **Sodium** 40mg, **Carbohydrates** 38g, **Dietary Fiber** 3g, **Protein** 2g
Dietary Exchanges: ½ Bread/Starch, 2 Fruit, ½ Fat

METRIC CONVERSION CHART

VOLUME MEASUREMENTS (dry)

1/8 teaspoon = 0.5 mL
1/4 teaspoon = 1 mL
1/2 teaspoon = 2 mL
3/4 teaspoon = 4 mL
1 teaspoon = 5 mL
1 tablespoon = 15 mL
2 tablespoons = 30 mL
1/4 cup = 60 mL
1/3 cup = 75 mL
1/2 cup = 125 mL
2/3 cup = 150 mL
3/4 cup = 175 mL
1 cup = 250 mL
2 cups = 1 pint = 500 mL
3 cups = 750 mL
4 cups = 1 quart = 1 L

VOLUME MEASUREMENTS (fluid)

1 fluid ounce (2 tablespoons) = 30 mL
4 fluid ounces (1/2 cup) = 125 mL
8 fluid ounces (1 cup) = 250 mL
12 fluid ounces (1 1/2 cups) = 375 mL
16 fluid ounces (2 cups) = 500 mL

WEIGHTS (mass)

1/2 ounce = 15 g
1 ounce = 30 g
3 ounces = 90 g
4 ounces = 120 g
8 ounces = 225 g
10 ounces = 285 g
12 ounces = 360 g
16 ounces = 1 pound = 450 g

DIMENSIONS

1/16 inch = 2 mm
1/8 inch = 3 mm
1/4 inch = 6 mm
1/2 inch = 1.5 cm
3/4 inch = 2 cm
1 inch = 2.5 cm

OVEN TEMPERATURES

250°F = 120°C
275°F = 140°C
300°F = 150°C
325°F = 160°C
350°F = 180°C
375°F = 190°C
400°F = 200°C
425°F = 220°C
450°F = 230°C

BAKING PAN SIZES

Utensil	Size in Inches/Quarts	Metric Volume	Size in Centimeters
Baking or Cake Pan (square or rectangular)	8×8×2	2 L	20×20×5
	9×9×2	2.5 L	23×23×5
	12×8×2	3 L	30×20×5
	13×9×2	3.5 L	33×23×5
Loaf Pan	8×4×3	1.5 L	20×10×7
	9×5×3	2 L	23×13×7
Round Layer Cake Pan	8×1½	1.2 L	20×4
	9×1½	1.5 L	23×4
Pie Plate	8×1¼	750 mL	20×3
	9×1¼	1 L	23×3
Baking Dish or Casserole	1 quart	1 L	—
	1½ quart	1.5 L	—
	2 quart	2 L	—